THE PCOD THYROID BOOK

RUJUTA DIWEKAR

THE PCOD THYROID BOOK

First published by Westland Publications Private Limited in 2016

Published by Westland Books, a division of Nasadiya Technologies Private Limited, in 2022

No. 269/2B, First Floor, 'Irai Arul', Vimalraj Street, Nethaji Nagar, Alapakkam Main Road, Maduravoyal, Chennai 600095

Westland and the Westland logo are the trademarks of Nasadiya Technologies Private Limited, or its affiliates.

ISBN: 9789395073110

10 9 8 7 6 5

Typeset by PrePSol Enterprises Private Ltd

Printed at Thomson Press India Private Limited

Contents

A Personal Note From Kareena Kapoor

Kareena Kapoor

"Oh God! I'm so busy today. I have no time to eat". The fastest selling excuse, easy to say and believe. Ever thought, 'I hardly ate anything today. I better feel and look thin.' Or, 'I am hardly eating. Why am I not losing weight?' Now my response to that is what my darling Rujuta Diwekar has taught me: "PLEASE EAT" or you are not going to loose weight.

Now, as an actress who works 18–20 hours a day, under gruelling circumstances (its −7°c sometimes, other times 50°c), shooting all night, playing and feeling a range of emotions – some days I have to cry a lot, and sometimes despite having my periods. I have to dance in the rain, trying to look beautiful and above all, trying to look and stay slim. But like I said come hail or storm, every 2–3 hours, my stomach makes a loud call of hunger, and like a good girl I attend to it. Now I am sure all the women reading this book probably don't have to dance in the rain, but definately have so many demands

→

On their time, its not that difficult, though, to slip in a slice of cheese, some peanuts or an apple in your handbag. Believe me, its all about the habit. It takes a week to cultivate a habit of stopping whatever your doing for just two minutes to grab a bite. I wouldn't give up my profession no matter what, its the most important thing in my life, but looking after my health and eating habits is a non-negotiable aspect of my life and its what keeps me going.

A very important aspect of us women are our ever changing hormones that lead to mood swings, acne, bloating and hair fall... we deal with a lot don't we?! Pregnancy cravings? oh! its all a part of it my lovely ladies. My advice is no need to scream "PANIC" when all these things happen. Just take out the time to EAT RIGHT. The day I come back from a long flight, I am extremely bloated, my hands and feet are swollen because of water retention, jet lag; lack of sleep and air pressure. But like rujuta says, lots of water and a home remedy of

Kareena Kapoor

ghar ka khana - some light dal, sabzi, and rice - and immediately re-starting my two-lovely diet, and the next day I instantly see the difference.

Women, if may say so, have an inherent ability to be beautiful. We just need to feel beautiful, and to feel gorgeous, remember, you have to eat your way to health, fitness and ultimately, "WEIGHTLOSS". What would I have done if I hadn't met and learned this from Rujuta? I am proud to eat and eat alot, despite being so busy.... It is the happiest feeling waiting for my next meal. It might not be bhajiyas and Vada Pav but who wants all that if I look like this and stay fit and healthy?

As I write this I am in Switzerland, enjoying the ripe fruits, berries and the yummy cheeses, the fresh milk and the avocado and aubergine sandwich in my hotel. Awesome! And I don't see myself putting on weight... Infact, I see myself, lovely ladies, "GLOWING"!

→

Is it the berries, is it Switzerland or was it the apple pie and vanilla Ice-Cream I had last night? Oops, Sorry RUJUTA! ☺

Much Love
To all,

Kareena Kapoor

Introduction

You think you should check your thyroid? If you haven't said it aloud, you have said it in your mind, and it's always in response to your body getting fat. It's like we almost don't think of our thyroid or our hormones in general if life is going our way, but we are quick to blame them when it is not. From obesity to bad skin, fertility to acne, mood swings to bloating, it's the bloody hormones. But are we really the victims of our hormones? Or are we the victims of our lifestyle?

The latest buzz in the bio-chemistry academe is to declare muscle, the skeletal muscle, that which moves on your command, as an endocrine organ. This is to really put the need to make lifestyle changes in perspective, give it the limelight and the long-due importance it deserves. Almost everyone is willing to pop a pill to regulate the thyroid or to get one's period, but how many are ready to work out even 150 minutes a week to regulate the thyroid and period cycle? Most of us accept (however incorrectly) that this pill is now a lifelong saathi, a partnership that will be broken only with death, but are we ready to partner with exercise till our last breath? Not quite. There's always something else to do — kids to be picked up, clothes to be laundered, hair to be blow-dried, etc. Then of course if it is something that requires a pill, it is taken more seriously by the family. Exercise on the other hand is considered a frivolous waste of time. Honestly, more people are ready to support your shopping instead of your exercise routine.

What we do know as scientific truth is that every cell in the body, especially the neurotransmitters, the glands and the hormones, respond beautifully to exercise just as they do to eating right. But how many of us will really commit to eating right? Most of us women are victims of what is called as chaotic eating. Chaotic eating is the exact opposite of regulated eating. Whether or not we will eat breakfast depends on what time we woke up or the children went to school. The chocolate box we finished last night was out of boredom and frustration, same with the vada pav that you ate the evening before. There is no plan, eating is an act of random happenings or accidents. Somehow though, if the period is late, thyroid is dull, etc., we never quite think it's the food, but that it's the hormones. Always, it's the hormones. But hormones are made out of the food we eat, and if your eating is more accidental than planned, then Allah Malik. Unless of course you decide to take charge, eh?

This book is about you taking charge, about you understanding that love and responsibility towards oneself is what you need to do daily. And sorry, but popping pills on time doesn't qualify either as love or responsibility, it stems out of fear and lack of accountability towards one's lifestyle. Food has the ability to heal, it is more powerful than any lab-made drug, and once you see food as the healer, the fear and fuss around food will disappear. Where fear about food ends, health begins. And with good health, the hormonal balance is restored. No, not with weight loss but with health. So first things first, forgive the doctor/dietician and everyone between who said that you must lose weight. Forgive even more the ones who said that you must lose five/ten or fifteen kilos to make your hormones better. Forgive, because they don't know what they say. They should have said 'gain health', not 'lose weight' for the desired effect, but darna and darana is unfortunately how the health business operates.

So let's look at the strategies that will help us and in turn our hormones. What can we do about our food, sleep, exercise and relationships that will make us feel good and lead a drug-free life. Read on: we made it easy for you and in this book is only what is relevant; nothing more, nothing less.

A recap of the four principles of eating right....

Principle 1: Eat something within the first ten-fifteen minutes of getting up. Tea/coffee should not be the first thing you have when you wake up. These stimulants will increase the blood pressure, heart rate, breathing rate and only end up stressing the body. In turn, the body will respond by hampering fat burning. On the other hand, if you eat something within the first fifteen minutes of getting up, blood sugar and energy levels increase, leading to an increase in metabolic rate and fat burning, and a decrease in acidity and bloating. You're less likely to overeat later and your blood sugars remain stable through the day. Basically, there's less chance of getting fat.

Principle 2: Eat every two hours. When you eat every two hours, your meals are more likely to be small. And when our body gets a small amount of calories at one time, they're utilised better and not stored as fat (because the body feels reassured with a regular intake of calories and nutrients), which means a flatter stomach. Also, you'll depend less on stimulants during the day.

Principle 3: Eat more when you're active and less when you are not. Your body's requirements change depending on your activity (mental or physical) levels, hormonal changes etc. Now, as you follow Principles 1 and 2, you'll get more in touch with the hunger signals your body is sending and when you feel like the need to eat more, do so. Eating more food when you're more active will make your body an efficient calorie burner, which will increase the metabolic rate of your body. This will make you stay energetic through the day and will help you lose fat more effectively.

Principle 4: Finish your last meal at least two hours prior to sleeping. An extension of Principle 3 — eat less post sunset and as your activities wind down. This way, most of your food is digested before you go to sleep, which will lead to a sound sleep, and leaves your body free to do its repair work.

...And the five basic rules to increase nutrient intake

1. Eat food that is prepared fresh, and eat it within three hours of cooking.
2. The smaller the number of people food is prepared for, the better its nutrient value.
3. Eat your vegetables and fruits whole; don't cut them or mash them into a juice.
4. Remain loyal to your genes: eat what you have been eating since childhood.
5. Eat what is in season. For example, mango in summer.

Rujuta Diwekar
Mumbai, October 2015

1

The Tamasha

Speak to any health professional in the country and they will tell you that men respond better to treatment than women, be it diabetes, malaria, weight loss or simply a pedicure. As women, we're guilty of supporting our men (father, brother, husband, son, father-in-law, son-in-law, brother-in-law) much more than we support ourselves or other women. The roots could be in the very fabric of our country, culture, tradition, religion, whatever, but we don't quite treat ourselves right or as equals. The most basic way in which we treat ourselves badly, is by denying ourselves the food we love, at the time we love and in quantities we love, and then of course to make things worse, we go about our life believing that our body owes it to us to stay toned, fit, lean and thin. Which is why this chapter even exists in this book, because we have bought into the tamasha, putting our health, body, nutrients, sleep, relationships and life itself at stake. When you read on, I want you to ask yourself if you identify with the behaviour patterns cited in the chapter, because I want you to give up thinking about your body as an object which deserves shame/criticism/something to be depressed over if it doesn't fit into some mould. I would actually sum it up with just two words — criticism kills. But if I had to write down reasons why women have such a hard time losing weight or why we behave so similar to the moon, reducing and gaining size every fortnight, here they are:

1. Always criticising your body
2. Running after results
3. Slave to the weighing scales
4. Obsessing over old jeans
5. Compromising on sleep

Let's look at each of them in detail with a real life example.

1. Always criticising your body

Real life example

Sarita walked in, looking fab in a black T-shirt and jeans, and got into an animated chat with Tejal, my nutritionist. They settled down in their chairs and began our usual exercise — discussing her diet recall and figuring out what went right, what went wrong, what needed to be changed and what would stay for the next two weeks. I had been listening to this conversation from my seat where I was writing some answers for an interview. Finally done, I walked out.

'Wow, Sarita, you look great!'

'Please! You always say that and you are the only one who says it.'

'Why? I'm sure Tejal told you the same thing as well.'

'Of course I did. You're really looking gorgeous, Sarita.'

'In fact, Sarita, you're looking so good, I'm going to make you some masala chai.'

'That's my weakness: I can never say no to masala chai. But, you know, I'm no longer waking up to chai in the morning; I eat a banana and actually feel good. I really never thought bananas would make me feel good! It's not so bad, not waking up to chai. But I'm still doing three cups, and am not able to cut it down.'

'Oh, come on, stop being harsh on yourself. You've cut down from eight to three cups, I think that's REALLY good, that's less than half your intake, ma'am.'

'Ya, but sometimes I do four, you know. Like today, you've asked me if I want chai. Now this will be my fourth cup and I don't have the willpower to say no.'

'Arrey, you come from a family of teachers or what?'

'Yes, my mom's one. Why?'

'Because you're so critical of your progress! You're just being nice to me by not refusing my offer to make chai; it's not that you lack willpower. You didn't exactly walk in begging for ek pyali chai, and you have cut down from eight cups of chai to three, and yet you are bothered that you have not been able to cut down on that one cup.'

'But my diet allows me only two cups.'

'Listen, it's okay. Your meal plan is a guideline, not a law that you cannot break. And you need to understand the logic behind cutting down on chai: it's to not suppress or kill appetite with a stimulant. And I think you're very much getting there, it's only been a month, come on!' I was patting her on her back.

'You really think I'm doing well?'

'Of course! I would never lie to you. I would think you are doing well even if you were down to six-seven cups from eight; every step in the right direction counts. Hello! What happened? The chai is so bad or what?'

Sarita was weeping, tears rolling down all the way to her chin. 'Nooo,' she shook her head; she was smiling through her tears, but she looked genuinely troubled. 'You know, just this morning, my husband complimented me on how good I was looking. He felt my stomach had gone down, my face was looking slimmer and my thighs were looking toned…'

'How cruel,' I joked.

'Please, I am already feeling bad. You know what I said to him?'

'No, but I can guess. You asked him to shut up.'

'No, worse. I gave him a big lecture on how he lacks integrity, how he just says things without meaning them, how I don't need his sympathy, and so what if I am fat, I am brilliant at what I do and how it's only a matter of time before I get thin so he should just stop giving me this crap.'

'Oh! Poor girl. I am so sorry. What did he say?'

'What could he say? He tried telling me that he really *could* see a difference, so I really lost it. I told him it's his fault that I'm fat, that he should have told me that I've been getting fatter. I've gained fifteen kilos in two years of being married, and this man said nothing!'

'You mean nothing critical?'

She stared at me with eyes that looked deadlier than a nuclear missile.

'You are very angry, na? He said some brilliant things to you this morning and you just resisted them with all your might. My guess is that you are only receptive to criticism — you know how to respond to it. But you are clueless about how to deal with appreciation, much less compliments.'

'You think so?'

'Absolutely. I told you that you were looking great, and Tejal said the same thing less than fifteen minutes ago, and your husband said it in the morning! Think about it.'

'Ya, actually even my team in office asked me if I was doing something because they said my face was looking better.'

'There you go. Then why are you having such a hard time accepting it?'

'Actually, it's the chai. If I don't follow my diet to perfection, I feel like I'm not doing it any justice and I'm not going to get anywhere....'

'Look Sarita, Tejal is not judging you for having a couple more cups of chai than your diet requires. It's not what Tejal thinks, it's what you think about yourself. You're judging yourself a bit too harshly. You haven't acknowledged how far you have come; your focus stays on how far you still have to go. It's a journey ya, it's not about getting to some place and getting to that place in less than four weeks or whatever. Seven-eight years of being an editor, seven-eight years of eight cups a day, and less than four weeks to overcome that habit and come down to three-four cups. Brilliant! Aren't you impressed with yourself? So, now Sarita, let's do it again.'

'What?'

'The compliment bit.' I went into rewind mode and did an action replay, walking back to my office, opening my door, looking at her and saying, 'Wow! You look great!'

This time, Sarita said, 'Thanks. I have been feeling great too....'

'Want a masala chai?'

'Yes!'

Like Sarita, most of us have to make the space in our head and heart to accept love and appreciation. On the one hand we strive for it, and on the other, we attack it if it crosses our path, or we are so indifferent to it that it rubs people the wrong way. Sarita had been married only two years and her husband still had the courage to compliment her. When women are married for longer, they almost train their husbands into submission. By that I mean they usually scold their husbands so much for saying nice things that they soon learn not to say much on this 'sensitive' topic. Women appear angry with their husbands, but they are usually just very angry with themselves. Very angry for not doing something to perfection, whatever that means. No matter what they do or what they achieve, they feel inadequate. **It's this feeling of inadequacy that we need to overcome, not our body weight.**

2. Running after 'results'

Real life example

I was getting an unsolicited motivational talk from a client, Deepika, who heads HR at an equity fund. 'Listen, this is my last hope. I have no face to show. I have wasted toooo much money on all this (weight loss fads and diet). Now you HAVE to give me results. You're the only one who can do that. If I don't see results, I just lose motivation. You can do it, Rujuta. You can give me results.'

'Wait a minute. What results?' I asked.

'What do you mean?' she shot back impatiently. 'Weight loss! And quick. I don't have much time. As it is, waiting to get an appointment with you wasted so much time. Now at least the results should be quick. I am sure you can do it. You charge a bomb, babe!'

This was not the first time I was hearing this. Nevertheless, I subjected her to my well-rehearsed answer: Just like happiness, good health cannot be bought.

'Can you elaborate on that?' Deepika cut me short. My team had nicknamed her 'Can you elaborate on that'. She had consistently repeated the phrase while we explained to her (in detail) the appointment procedure, waiting time, what to expect while on a package, how she could take these two months forward.... Would you like a glass of water? Can you elaborate on that?

So I did elaborate. 'Good health is priceless, it cannot be bought. You need to work at it constantly. It needs effort. Your effort. Enough effort to eventually make it effortless. You are paying me to educate you about good eating habits and to work with you to find ways to eat right given your hectic schedule. Which means that you're not paying me two rupees (or any other denomination) per gram of weight lost.'

'So? Does that mean that I have wasted my money?'

'Can you elaborate on that?' (Wow!! I had managed to win the competition in my office. I had actually asked 'Can you elaborate on that', 'Can you elaborate on that?')

'I need results! Weight loss.'

'I'm sorry, then yes, you *are* wasting your money. Weight loss should come free. You shouldn't need to pay anything for it.'

'Elaborate on that?'

'Okay, diarrhoea and dysentery can result in weight loss. You don't have to pay to get diseases. The latest and most exotic one is swine flu. Swine flu can give good results. Results = weight loss. I can't. What I will essentially do is help you gain weight.'

'WHAT??'

'Sit down Deepika, and let me elaborate. Have you seen the movie *Kuch Kuch Hota Hai*?'

'Yes. But what does it have to do with anything?'

'You know what you need in your body so that kuch kuch happens? Metabolically active muscle tissue. Muscle occupies very little volume in your body compared to fat and has the property to contract and send electrical impulses. You can grow denser muscle and a better network of nerves around it if you work out regularly, eat right, sleep right and think right. The diet plan that we come up with together will pretty much encourage you to avoid diet or food accidents, take to regular exercise and have a regular sleep/waking-up pattern — all of which will make you gain weight. Denser muscles and denser bones = weight gain.'

'Okay, I am kind of getting a grip on this. Tell me more.'

'Cool, so we are on the same page now (I love dishing out corp lingo to corp types). Deepika, a gain in lean body weight — that's the weight of your bones and muscles — is like reversing the process of ageing. As age progresses and inactivity sets in, our muscles shrink and our bones get hollow or brittle, so you lose lean body weight (LBW) and that all-important ability to keep your fat stores burning. End result? Total gain in body weight as a result of weight loss.

'Now if you equate results with weight loss, then it just makes things difficult for you. You will put an effort into eating right, working out, regularising bedtime and stuff so you will look better, feel better, your body volume will shrink, everybody around you will start telling you that you have lost weight and you will end up feeling stronger and more energetic than ever before. But then if these changes don't come with a shift in the weighing scales you feel like a loser, because you still don't have the "results" you signed up for.'

'So now what?'

'Now we just work at what is within our reach and forget about "results". Especially about putting a deadline for results. Once your body receives the right nutrients at the right time, it will start prioritising the repair work that it wants to bring about in your system. It's best that you leave this to inner wisdom and not interfere with this process. So if your body wants to take care of depleted nutrient stores, optimise hormonal response, grow denser bones, teeth, nails or hair, you let it be. You should feel confident that your body will never work against you. It will continue to drop fat stores through this process, but just because this is not reflecting on the scales it doesn't mean that it's not happening. See, we are often unaware of the fact that we are breathing or that the earth is moving around the sun, but just because we are not conscious of the process, it doesn't mean that it's not happening. It's still happening. You are breathing, right?'

'Ya, I just never thought of it this way. But it makes sense. So my money is safe. Thank you.'

The elaboration had ended, but I added, 'So the "takeaway" here is that weight loss is not proof of fat loss or better health.'

'But how do I evaluate my progress? Will it ever, finally, eventually lead to weight loss or are people like me doomed to stay fat?'

'Well, as long as you *feel* light, know that you are getting lighter on the fat stores. See Deepika, learning to eat right is about dropping tension that you carry in your mind and body, and not about dropping weight. **So if you feel lighter in body and mind, you no longer need the weighing scale to validate the fact that you are on track.** But do yourself a favour and don't take it up like a project that you need to deliver within a timeline. Be as compassionate with your body as it has been with you. Heard this song? The one Kamal Haasan sings from the roof of a bus — *Jitne bhi tu karle sitam, has has ke sahenge hum, yeh pyaar na hoga kum, sanam teri kasam....* So motivation to treat the body well should be unconditional. The love your body has shown you is unconditional no matter what you put her through — starvation, late-night binges, fad diets, all of it ya. She stood by you through everything. Payback time now.'

The gym punishment

There's a girl in the gym I go to who walks in at 6 a.m. (the gym opens at 5.30) and leaves at 9.45 — that's 9.45 at night. And that too when she's practically pushed out by the trainers because the gym closes at 10 p.m. Maybe it's partly to do with her being an aspiring actor and wanting to network in the gym, but a lot of us struggling with weight loss do tend to stay in the gym for two, two-and-a-half hours at a stretch. The truth is, anything more than a sixty-minute workout will lead to a loss of muscle tissue; this leads to a lower metabolic rate, which means that you're burning less fat through the day. Basically, exercising for more than an hour actually defeats the purpose of exercise — the exact opposite of what you're aiming for takes place. It's not a maths equation where, if you lose y amount of calories in an hour, you'll lose y x 2 calories if you work out for two hours. There's a lot of chemistry, biology and biomechanics involved. Consider what part of your body is taking the strain of over-exercise, what fuel you're burning, fat or muscle. Is it actually helping your blood circulation or making your body weaker?

Exercising is a way of loving your body, not punishing it. And spending more than an hour in the gym is like two-timing someone you love. Cheating on someone is never easy on the mind, body or senses, so it's no surprise that if you overexercise, your body will show it — and not in the way you want. The point of exercise is that you should look like you've worked out, like you're toned, whether you're in your work clothes, saree or a salwar kameez. Instead, you'll have the kind of body where people will ask you if you've been ill.

3. Slave to the weighing scales

'Don't look at me like that,' said Praveen.

'No, I'm not looking at you. (Actually, I was glaring.) Do you really think I'm ever going to ask you mera wajan kyon nahi kam ho raha hai?'

He smiled sheepishly and shook his head. I had signed up for personal training with Praveen and he was putting me through the rigmarole of checking my body weight. Why was I giving him a dirty look? Because on three different weighing scales in the gym, my weight had gone from 52.5 to 51 and finally 50 kilos. 'Yippee, I have lost weight!' should have been my delighted response.

Instead I was going into a zone of 'why do women practically put their life on hold for this dumb thing' and other 'how we make a mountain out of a molehill' issues. The problem was, I couldn't afford to do that. I was running late and had a workout to finish.

There are two *big* problems with checking body weight: 1) The weighing scales are *never* accurate. 2) And this is the bigger one — body weight is in *no* way an indicator of your health, fitness or beauty. I think we pretty much understand the first problem. My clients often inform me how they weigh X on their bathroom scales, Y on their gym scales and Z on their doctor's scales. To add a little more fun to their lives, they want to check their weight on my scales. When I say I don't have one, they demand to know what kind of a dietician's office is this if it doesn't even have a weighing scale. Instead of answering them, I ask if they'd like some jasmine chai. 'Jasmine tea, by the way, is a great relaxant. A relaxed state of mind is imperative for the success of the meal plan that I will suggest post the chai.' My standard line.

When you are relaxed, you generally don't behave harshly with yourself. I mean, as women, we have been brainwashed into always being nice to others, especially after marriage, but we're never told not to behave 'rudely' to ourselves. So we are all guilty of doing tons of emotional atyachar on ourselves daily. But when we feel relaxed we are willing to go easy on ourselves. So no weighing scales but jasmine chai. Tumhare paas kya hai? Mere paas jasmine chai hai!

Okay, jokes apart, families have been broken, money has been laundered, health has been lost and the body has been put through near-death experiences — all to see some elusive number on a weighing scale. One of my clients lost her mother due to a complication post liposuction (she wanted to lose weight quickly for her son's wedding). Her story almost killed me. I mean, what's wrong with us? Whom are we trying to please, and at what cost? I couldn't have possibly lost 2.5 kilos in less than thirty seconds — that's about the time I took to hop from one scale to another. And yet I know that it's standard practice in the gym for women to get themselves checked on all three weighing scales so they have yet another thing to whine about. Oh! Only three hundred grams? What, still sixty-seven?

Let's look at it this way — just because you have never had a showdown with your mother-in-law, is it safe to assume that you love her? No? There you go. The number on the weighing scale is as much an indicator of health, fitness and beauty as the absence of a showdown is an indicator of love. Or standing first in class an indicator of smartness. Even schools are now adopting more holistic and inclusive methods to assess the progress of children —

shouldn't our fitness/weight-loss plans do the same? What are these holistic ways? Actually, you will just *know* whether you are doing well or not; you won't need a scale to tell you. I bet you're thinking that this whole 'you-will-just-know' thing is too out there. Okay, let's try and put it in words:

1. Are you waking up fresher?
2. Have your cravings decreased?
3. Are you feeling lighter in your body?
4. Are you feeling inspired to exercise?
5. Are your nails growing faster than the scheduled manicure appointment?
6. Is your skin feeling and looking fresher? Have the blemishes and acne decreased?
7. Do you feel like catching up with friends/family more often?
8. Do you feel like shopping (for clothes for yourself)?
9. Are you feeling hungry often?
10. Are you smiling often?

If you answered in affirmative to most questions, congrats, you are in love with yourself. Tougher than being in love with your partner/parents/children/pet, etc. And you are also on the way to losing fat the right way. The right way being the one that is doable, sustainable and enjoyable. You have set yourself free from moronic activities like checking your body weight and are ready to enjoy life to its fullest.

So now what should we do with our weighing scales? THROW them away. And if your raddi wala is willing to buy it, sell it, add Rs 1000 to that amount from my behalf and donate the money to a good cause. It will make you feel lighter. Weighing scales belong to a bygone era, not to the woman of today. So don't let your happiness or sadness depend on a number, move on. There's more to life.

Now what's the jasmine chai connection? If you've answered 'yes' to most of the questions above, you are actually experiencing a fairly good degree of calmness. A calm mind mobilises fatty acids and uses body fat as the most preferred fuel (to sustain metabolism). This way it spares the lean body tissues, keeping you not just 'light' on stress but also on the scales. Now you know why I choose the chai and not the scales.

'I need something drastic right now!'

'Eat all the time? Eat according to the four principles? You must be kidding! Look at my size. I am ninety-eight kilos and just two years ago I was more than a hundred. You have no idea what all I have done to lose weight: enema, starvation, lime shots, dudhi juice, needles poked in my body, puked dinner after eating it, worked out till I fainted, didn't eat till I fainted and now you want me to *eat?'*

'Why don't you want to? You prefer fainting or throwing up food to sensible eating?' I asked.

'No, it's not that. I am prepared to die to eat normally, but I think before that I must knock off at least twenty-thirty kilos. Once I knock that off, trust me I will eat whatever you ask me to and as many times as you want.'

'Great, then what are we doing right now? If you feel that you must be doing "drastic" things to knock off "initial weight", this is the wrong place.'

'Don't say that. I have tried everything.'

'That's exactly my point Aliya, you have tried everything and most of it — in fact all of it — was drastic. You have fluctuated, gaining all the weight you lost, and worse, yo-yoed that way several times. Seriously, I think the most "DRASTIC" thing that you can do now is EAT. And eat as normally as you would if you were ten/twenty/fifty kilos lighter.'

What I hope I made Aliya understand is that loving your body, totally and unconditionally accepting it, and being willing to nourish it with good food is the only way to lose fat and improve muscle tone, or as it's popularly called, 'lose weight'. These drastic measures that we adopt to lose the 'initial weight' only lead to drastic damages to the body, the worst being a perpetually shifting body weight. And, much like the Indo-Pak peace talks, where you take one step forward and two steps backward, you always land up in a situation worse than where you started off.

4. Obsessing over old jeans

'Throw them out.'

Parul looked startled. 'Come on, Rujuta. Kuch toh marker hona chahiye. Don't stand on the weighing scale, don't go by the weighing scale, so what do I go by? I should have my old jeans for that no?' It was our first meeting and Parul had gone gaga about *Don't Lose Your Mind, Lose Your Weight* for the first fifteen minutes, but then came down to business. She wanted to lose weight and had thoroughly understood that she shouldn't 'hold herself to ransom' with the weighing scales.

'So are you looking at an alternative place to hold yourself to ransom?'

'Am I really? That sounds terrible.'

'Ya, but I think that's exactly what you are doing.'

'No, Vaishali said she did the two-month programme with you and doesn't know how much weight she lost, but she now fits into jeans she wore in college. And that's why I joined. I have kept my jeans from high school too, right in the front of my wardrobe to motivate myself. I HAVE to fit into them. It's size twenty-eight, I am now wearing thirty-six (sad face).'

'So for how long have you tangoed them in front of your wardrobe for motivation?'

'I got them in '95, so I've had them forever now, but honestly, it's only after Vaishali showed off that she can fit into her college jeans that I brought mine out.'

'And have you lost weight in these six-seven months?'

'No, but I booked an appointment with you, so that's a good start.'

'Okay, so now throw them out.'

'Why?'

'Because I want to make things easy for you (and for myself). Look, staring at jeans that are now almost from the Stone Age makes us feel ancient and that really doesn't help. Our body changes, it's inevitable, you've got to make peace with it. All you need to figure out is how much (and how many) of those changes are natural and how much of it is just circumstantial.'

'Circumstantial bole ga toh?'

'Bole ga toh, enforced. Matlab, see, what were you eating in '95? What were your activities in '95? What were your stresses in '95? Where were you staying in '95? What were your responsibilities in '95? How much time did you have for yourself in '95? Were you exercising in '95?

Was it your responsibility to ensure that everybody in the household is eating and on time?'

'Yes, the circumstances under which I had a waist of twenty-eight were SOO different.'

'There you go. So don't put those jeans there; simply figure out how much of '95 you can recreate, that will bring you closer to that slim-fit, narrow waist twenty-eight jeans. Can you spare at least half the time to exercise? At least eat half as often? Can you cut back on your current stresses, at least a bit? Can you be a little more responsible towards yourself — at least half the sense of responsibility that you have towards your kids, husband, in-laws, keeping a clean kitchen, wardrobe, etc.?'

'Come on ya! It's not just that!! Okay, I mean I have been kind of a kitchen goddess and all that. So okay I own up to it. But let's be real. I was twenty-four in '95. I am touching forty now. Age is a factor too. Let's blame age. No?'

'No. Let's thank age. It teaches us — if we are willing to learn — that hanging on to old jeans doesn't help, giving up on them does. Age only means body changes, it doesn't mean it deteriorates. Whether it changes for the better or for worse is up to you. Kareena looks younger and sexier today than she did five years ago.'

'Ya, she is gorgeous. But please, she is just about thirty!'

'Okay, how about Saif?'

'Okay ya, he definitely looks hotter by the day. And now that you say it, even Shah Rukh tweeted that he can do more with his body now than he did fifteen years ago.'

'See, there you go! I say that about my body too. My mind, my body, both are calmer, stronger, better than they were fifteen years ago.'

'Ya, you're thirty-something too.'

'Yes, but I am talking of fifteen years irrespective of age; and I see that with all my clients no matter what their age. Should I tell you the secret? Ready for this?'

Deep breath, eyes closed, 'Yes.'

'Here goes: treat your body like it's not yours, treat it like it's somebody else's and you have it on rent for a while. Puzzled? Think about it as something really expensive that a friend has lent you and you can use it to get all you want and desire. You only have to look after it in return. It's like, if I give you my car, you would drive it at least ten times more carefully than how you drive your car. Drive it slower over speed-breakers, return it with a full petrol tank, have the right amount of air in the tyres, not jump signals, etc.?'

'Ya…'

'With our own car, the minute we think "this is mine", that sense of ownership — instead of making us more responsible — makes us irresponsible. We will do things that we know are clearly wrong, that we would never do with someone else's. So get out of the age-old "age excuse". **Use your body like a "single hand-driven Parsi-owned car"**. Get more responsible towards it, at least with things that you clearly know are wrong. Those things that you would not do with someone else's body — starving it/over-exercising it/making a couch potato out of it/stressing it with non-issues/kicking it with caffeine/clogging it with trans fat and processed food. Staying irresponsible with food and exercise and refusing to give up on old jeans is like full-on torture, ya.

'Also, the fact is, as you progress in the journey of getting leaner, fitter and more responsible towards your body, you don't just drop to a twenty-eight size. You get there centimetre by centimetre, dropping from thirty-six to thirty-four to thirty-two and further down. And you should celebrate the process, the journey, not the "arrival". The worst thing you can do as you progress from thirty-six to thirty-two is feel bad because you are not twenty-eight yet. Sensible and responsible is the name of the game, babe. As you move down sizes, you should jump in joy and punch your fist in the air. Better than yesterday and will be even better tomorrow. Just treat it like somebody else's body, and then buy new jeans for it after you have forsaken the sense of ownership over it.'

5. Compromising on sleep

Sound sleep is the most essential, integral, non-negotiable aspect of losing body fat. I can't overemphasise the importance of a restful, peaceful sleep. It's the one thing that you must have if you want a narrower waist, flatter stomach and toned body.

Real life example

It was just over 7 p.m. and Nandini was looking washed-out and dead tired. It was our first meeting. She had woken up at 8 a.m., eaten nothing, drunk a cup of coffee and gone to the gym. Had 'grabbed a toast and egg-whites' for breakfast and drunk two-three cups of tea and one black coffee during back-to-back meetings till afternoon. Then she'd had a meeting with her chef, tasting and testing some yummy dishes he had made, thus overeating because the dishes were too delicious and anyway, 'I was so hungry by that time'. Then she had rushed through traffic, screamed at her driver, instructed the cook at home about what to make for dinner for saab, ordered the maid to make sandwiches for the kids and wash laundry that had been hanging in the bathroom for three days, also called the AC guy to get the vents cleaned. Then, as her driver parked the car, she'd rushed up to my office and profusely apologised for being fifteen minutes late. I tried to say, 'Chalta hai', but I don't think she heard. She was yawning and collapsing on my sofa. She wasn't dying or going into a coma, she was just dead tired and very sleepy.

A lot of 'career women' (a term I can't fully understand) have days that are just as hectic (sorry, normal) as Nandini's. Unis-bees ka farak. (Some of us are becoming the men we wanted to marry – Gloria Steinem.) So I had the task of telling her important things when I thought she was listening, which I was about to realise was never. She was either yawning or talking or saying, 'Sorry, I have to take this', before answering her phone.

How do I know her recall for the day? Because she had emailed it to me from her phone, in the car, while on her way to my office. The day before her appointment, I had been informed that, despite numerous calls, sms-es and emails, we were yet to receive the recall of her diet for the last three days. As a policy, we cancel appointments if we haven't received a client's recall, so I'd got hers last minute, as 'damage control', but only after we had given her office and her a lot of grief.

As Nandini sat on my sofa, yawning, I felt at a loss for words and was kind of overwhelmed by all the activity around me. Instinctively I wanted to put a blanket on her tired body, a pillow under the overworked head and let her nap for a while. But of course that was 'not done'. As I tried to say something, the phone rang again. It was her daughter on the line (she had a policy: if it's a call from her son or daughter, take it, no matter what, where, etc.), complaining that the chutney was too teekha and that Swati (the maid) had once again put Simla mirch in the sandwich. 'Okay baby, I'll get it sorted out. Give the phone to Swati,' she said while signalling 'two minutes' with her fingers to me. 'Swati, kitne baar bolna padega? Baby ko Simla mirch nahi, that's only for Baba. Aur chutney kyon teekha hua hai? Abhi usme thoda nimbu dalo aur please thoda dhyan rakho.'

Whoa!! 'Can we put the phone on silent?' I suggested when it rang again.

'Just this one call ... Ya love, it's the eighteenth,' she said to her husband, and then, to me, 'Okay, I will put it on silent now.'

I was already feeling sapped of energy, and I had only spent a little over ten minutes with Nandini. 'Wow! I think you're going to go home and CRASH!' I said.

She smirked. 'That would be a sweet dream for me RD, if I could hit the pillow and sleep.'

'Why? You look like you're ready to sleep right now.'

'Ya, I am feeling sleepy and dead tired right now. In fact, that's how I feel through the day, but sleep for me is nothing less than a nightmare!'

'Why?'

'See I go back home and then there are hajjar things to do and I want to spend some good, quality time with my kids. And then by about 9.30 my kids go to bed and I go to my bedroom to finally get some "me time" and also to spend some time with my husband. I think we spend less than three hours with each other from Monday to Friday. So till about 10.30 – 11 I watch TV or I'm on my laptop checking emails and stuff. After that I try hard to go to bed, to sleep, sleep, sleep, but I lie down for hours, WIDE awake. I think about duniya bhar ka kaam, when all I want to do is SLEEP. It's such a struggle, I can't tell you. I feel like I'm cursed; you will have everything in life — money, husband, kids, career everything — but, hey, you won't be able to sleep. Finally, at around 3.30 – 4 a.m., after having raided the fridge, and gone to the bathroom at least five times, I doze off for a bit. Then, of course, I have to wake up by 7 to get the kids ready for school, Viren comes back from squash and I have to go to the gym to work my fat ass off and then to work. It's a battleground man, full throttle. Always sleepy, and never able to actually sleep'.

'For how long have you had this problem with sleep? When was the last time you slept well and woke up fresh?'

'I can't remember. Must be long, long ago. I think I have had this issue now for more than thirteen years!'

'What?'

'Yeah, babe. Okay, are you telling me what to eat? I have to rush back.'

'You don't need a diet babe, you need a BREAK!'

Are you kidding me? I can't afford to take one.'

'*You're* kidding me. I think what you can't afford is to go without sleep like this. And it's only going to get you fat.'

'You know I slog my ass off at the gym. I want to slap all the skinny bitches I see there. So much of working out and you saw my recall? I hardly eat. (I wanted to interject with, Ya, this recall won't do and stuff, but there was no chance.) So if I am not losing weight with no food and phatte workouts, how am I going to lose weight by *sleeping?*'

Lack of sleep (among many other things) screws up your recovery from exercise and life. Exercise 'works' on the basic premise that you will recover from the damage caused to the body while working out. If there's no recovery, fat burning comes to a grinding halt, exposing you to injuries, hormonal imbalances (hypothyroid, insulin resistance), digestion issues, mood swings and even panic attacks.

Now, just like love, money can't buy sleep either. So to sleep you really need to loosen up and take a chill pill. (I didn't use the words 'chill pill' with her. I know from experience that most moms hate that term. Especially if you say the word 'mom' immediately before or after 'chill pill'.) Essentially you need to review your priority list. Put yourself (and sleep and REST) at the top of your priority list. Yes, yes, yes we need to take it easy. It's anyway too difficult to achieve anything superlative when you are dog tired, and even if you do (luck by chance), it's almost impossible to derive any joy out of it.

So if your senses are being pulled in several different directions — bai, bachche, kaam, dhaam and the likes — they don't get a chance to get centred or to withdraw from these assumed responsibilities. (By assuming responsibility I mean Nandini's daughter could easily have removed the Simla mirch from the sandwich herself or told the maid to; the husband could have checked whether it's the eighteenth or twentieth or whatever, etc.) When the senses can't withdraw themselves from external stimuli, rest or sleep is hard to come by. Deep or peaceful sleep is when you experience 'nothing', and for this you should be blessed with the ability to withdraw.

Now for women who are pulled in all directions all day, winding down in front of the TV while lying on the bed is a strict NO-NO. You can do without knowing what Anandi, Ecchha, Carrie Bradshaw or Sagarika Ghose are up to. Worse still, you get to watch your partner while he surfs channels on the TV, doing nothing and saying nothing. Seriously, if you want to rest, switch off and sleep.

Switch off the TV, lights, BB, Mac; light a nice non-toxic, calming agarbatti/scented candle or oil; wash your feet in warm water; apply a drop of ghee/til oil to the soles of your feet; and then lie on your bed, pull a soothing chaddar over yourself and experience 'nothing'. You will wake up ready to experience everything.

And you still want to watch TV? Cool, just move it to another room. Watch it, and when you've had enough, switch it off. The slimmer the TV and the closer it is to your bed, the bigger your waist and the further your navel is from your spine. More on Nandini's story and the damage that the lack of sleep can cause to your hormones and metabolism later (Chapter 2). For now, just move the TV out.

Forgive, forget, forward

So you've just started on a diet, got stuck somewhere and can't eat Meal 4. You decide, chalo, today's diet is anyway gone, let me skip Meal 5 as well and have Diet Pepsi and pizza for Meal 6. Or you got up late on Wednesday and you had a conference call on Thursday morning, so you couldn't work out on both days, and you think, I might as well not do Friday since this week's workout plan has been bad anyway. The thing to do in both these cases, is not get disheartened. If you skipped Meal 4, it's okay, it happens. Eat your Meal 5 and 6 as if you've had Meal 4. You need to forgive yourself for these occasional slips. If you know you have a con call in the morning, go work out in the evening, or go to sleep the previous day knowing you will miss your workout. Don't feel guilty.

Look at the way we learnt to walk. We fell numerous times in the process, but did we feel bad, judge ourselves, and just continue to crawl for the rest of our lives? No, we continued to consistently work at it. Of course, one thing we can't overlook is that our support group at that point was strong: our parents and the people around us constantly encouraged us through the process. But, most importantly, we didn't judge ourselves. The same with your diet and workout plan. Falling now and then is part of the natural learning curve — an essential part in fact — and it's not unnatural. But you have to keep moving ahead and continue to follow it. Forgive and forget won't work — you have to forgive, forget and move forward.

2

Hypothyroid

What is it? How does it function?

Now before we start talking about the thyroid gland and how/why it malfunctions, this is what you should know:

a) There isn't enough known about the exact working mechanism of the thyroid.
b) But there is enough to know that in no way will it interfere with your 'weight loss' plans (so stop blaming your thyroid before reading further).
c) Nutrition (actually lack of it) plays a huge role in disturbing the thyroid.
d) Stress (actually our inability to deal with it — blame it on poor eating again) can disturb it too.
e) Lack of sensible exercise (and no, walked in London/mall-hopped in Dubai/took stairs in office/sat in the sauna don't count as exercise) compounds the problem.
f) Now I know you will love this one: being a woman does put you at an increased risk of thyroid malfunction.
g) Pregnancy and menopause put you at a higher risk.
h) Lack of sleep, recovery and rest irritate the thyroid further.

Okay, enough of the layman stuff. Let's get into the jargon now.

The thyroid gland is shaped like a beautiful butterfly and is in your neck, in front of your wind pipe, just below the 'Adam's apple'. Its function is to produce a group of hormones, collectively called as the 'thyroid hormone'. The thyroid hormone regulates your body's metabolism and the way your body utilises carbs, fat and protein for growth, development and energy in every single cell of the body, not to forget temperature regulation. It also helps release catecholamines like dopamine, the 'feel good' hormone. And it influences every other hormone in the body because, obviously, everything in our body is interlinked. So if one of our hormones doesn't work at its peak efficiency, then all our other hormones, like the growth hormone, insulin, estrogen, etc., suffer too. And because they are suffering, it takes a toll on our neurotransmitters and enzymes. And then because our neurotransmitters and enzymes are feeling out of sync, our vitamin and mineral synthesis starts taking a beating. And because the vitamin and mineral synthesis is not up to the mark, our fat metabolism, calcium absorption, sleeping patterns, mood stabilisers, alertness, everything suffers. Get the picture? Our health is like the palace you made with a deck of cards. You remove one card or alter its position, the entire palace looks like it's going to collapse; it may not collapse immediately, but it becomes more vulnerable for sure. Then you do something completely unrelated to the palace, like moving the chair next to the table or bang the door of a room, and *phrrr,* your palace is down.

Chalo, let's get back to the main players in this game. The main thyroid hormones are t4 and t3. Thyroxine or t4 is considered as the precursor (gets converted) to the more active triiodothyronine or t3 and is present in much larger amounts and has a larger half-life than t3 (i.e. it sustains itself longer in the body). Now your thyroid gland is controlled by another gland called the pituitary gland, which is the size of a peanut and is located at the base of the brain. More specifically, the anterior pituitary produces the Thyroid Stimulating Hormone (TSH), which tells the thyroid gland to produce t4 and t3. The pituitary gland gets the signal to produce TSH from another gland called the hypothalamus, which is inside our brain. So the hypothalamus will produce the TSH-releasing hormone (TRH), which will signal to the pituitary to stimulate the thyroid to produce t4, t3 by secreting TSH. Phew!

Let's recap:

TRH →	TSH →	t4 →	t3
Released by hypothalamus, inside the brain	Released by pituitary	The thyroid hormone is secreted, in the presence of iodine + tyrosine, a protein	The active thyroid hormone — triiodothyronine

Now once TSH is released, the thyroid needs iodine and tyrosine to produce t4 and t3. Iodine is a mineral that is very crucial for the body because it's involved in making thyroid hormones, which is central to your body's metabolism. I mean, we all keep talking about sluggish metabolism or have hopes of raising our basal metabolic rate (BMR), but how many of us talk about consuming adequate iodine? Without adequate iodine in your diet, you are fighting a losing battle against fat loss.

Tyrosine, the protein that iodine bonds with to make your thyroid hormone, is a non-essential amino acid whose levels in our body are controlled by an essential amino acid L-phenylalanine. So again, without adequate intake of protein and without the right ratios of essential to non-essential amino acids, the metabolic rate won't rise. Are you getting the story?

Tyrosine along with iodine makes thyroid hormones = normal functioning of thyroid hormones, crucial to optimise metabolism = metabolism that works well = fat that burns well = well, you simply can't afford to be fussy or faddish about your diet.

Okay, okay. It's really not as simple as tyrosine + iodine = thyroid hormone. Many things, enzymes, amino acids, neurotransmitters, vitamins, minerals are involved in the process of bringing iodine and tyrosine together. The chief ones being vitamin B6, vitamin C, manganese, and the enzyme iodine peroxidase (all enzymes are protein based).

So as the thyroid hormones pass through your blood, your brain measures their amount, and if it feels that the amount is low, it will signal the pituitary to secrete a higher amount of TSH. There, you just got declared as having 'hypothyroidism'. No, not by your brain, by your blood test. For the brain is only trying to help you and not label you. A higher amount of TSH is being secreted to help you produce adequate amounts of t4 and therefore t3. It also works the reverse way: when the blood has more than adequate thyroid hormones, the levels of TSH drop.

The family doctor

The good doc is fast disappearing, being replaced by the 'specialist'. You have a stomach ache? Go straight to the gastroenterologist. Got a headache? Straight to the neurologist. Backache? See an orthopaedic. With the 'family doctor' disappearing and losing credentials (in some cases, rightly so), an important link in our health care system is missing. Take the example of high TSH levels (above normal) along with normal t3 and t4 or a high-fasting blood sugar along with normal post-lunch levels. A 'specialist' who spends five minutes (or less) with you in the consulting room is far less likely to make the right diagnosis than a GP who has watched you grow up, knows what your parents' blood pressure/ fasting sugars were like, and has met your husband/children, knows your job profile, working hours, etc. A lot of times, in fact most of the time, you need more than a blood test, X-ray, MRI, etc. to make the right decision about a line of treatment.

Sometimes, plain stress, lack of rest, a bad relationship, frequent flying, the death of a loved one, shifting, change in climate, diet, exercise, can manifest themselves as high TSH or high fasting sugars. What you need then is a professional who is willing to spend time with you understanding the discrepancies in your blood levels and someone who has a fair understanding of your genetic predisposition (beyond the obvious question of 'anybody in family with thyroid/blood pressure/diabetes?') and current changes in lifestyle. A good family doctor fits the bill and can work as a buffer, protecting you from unnecessary medicines and procedures. But then, family doctor, specialist or super specialist, patronising the right and credible doctor is your responsibility. So make sure your doctor (whatever hierarchy or qualification) encourages you to ask questions and answers them patiently in words that you understand. We don't want to pay through our noses for illegible prescriptions written on a shabby piece of paper, but we will pay through our noses, ear, mouth everything to be reassured and well taken care of when sick. Know that it's within your right to be informed about your 'condition'. Know that consent can be obtained and risks of procedures or drugs can be understood only when you are empowered with information, not when you sign on a piece of paper that's called a 'waiver'.

Thyroid and weight loss

Amongst the most frequent questions that I am asked by women who are overweight or those who have 'unsuccessfully' been on many diet plans is, 'Do you think I have a thyroid problem?' Or then there is this final declaration: 'I don't think I can lose weight because I have a thyroid problem'. Or else confessions: 'My doctor/dietician says I won't lose weight because of my thyroid'. And worse: 'I hope I get hyperthyroid so that I can lose weight'!!

So here's what you should really know: if you believe that you have a 'thyroid problem' and therefore must accept a 'weight problem', then you have simply been misled. There is absolutely no reason whatsoever for you to believe that you are doomed or that the body weight won't budge because of a 'thyroid problem' or 'thyroid'. Way too many emails in my inbox have read: 'Hi, your book is great. But I have a thyroid problem so is there some hope for me?' Or: 'Do you think you can still help me?'

Typically, this is what my answer reads like:

Hi,

Thanks for writing in.

Of course the four principles will help you too.

Eating right and working out regularly will help you support your thyroid function and fat metabolism.

Do keep me updated on your progress and stay in touch.

All the best.

Rujuta

You shouldn't feel disheartened about having a 'thyroid'. If you read the first few paragraphs, you will know we all have the gland and should thank it profoundly for all the functions that it carries, not the least of which is fat burning. And calling it a 'thyroid problem', puhleeese! First of all, know that while you were gestating in your mother's womb and were only about three to four weeks old, the thyroid gland was formed under your tongue. Soon it started helping you grow and most importantly started developing your brain, making it sharp, alert, logical, analytical and reasonable. All this work, so that you can function and think 'normally'. The name 'thyroid' is derived from Greek, and it means shield. So the thyroid gland has shielded you from growth and development abnormalities when you were still in your mother's womb, it's been with you since week four. And then by the eighteenth-twentieth week, it also started producing its own t3, t4 so that it could shield your mother from over-activating her thyroid. Now tell me how the ever-giving, nurturing, shielding thyroid must feel when we blame it singularly for our weight gain. We really are so ungrateful! And so stupid too, to feel that all our problems will be resolved only if the thyroid works well.

Our body is interlinked; just one organ/hormone/muscle/bone/nerve/cell is not causing a problem to our body or life. In fact, our way of life is causing a problem to the entire body and it is simply getting manifested in one of our already overworked body parts. More often than not, our 'problem area' also happens to be the area which has done maximum work for us or has shielded us against all the 'problems' our lifestyle, stress, diet, exercise, relationships, working hours, etc. have caused.

Will it expose me to other curses?

Yes. Leave a thyroid without support (and I mean SUPPORT, not a pill) long enough and it will lead to problems in many other areas. The most susceptible ones are high triglycerides levels (circulating fat which at high levels puts you at risk of developing heart disease), diabetes, sleeplessness, painful periods, constant fatigue, low bone density, low vitamin D levels, and of course weight gain. Sometimes it may even lead to PCOD, high blood pressure ... the list really is endless.

And what exposes me to hypothyroidism?

More women than men suffer from hypothyroidism, and the reason is the big hormonal events that we go through in our life, mainly pregnancy and menopause.

During pregnancy, the hormonal balance in our body shifts and our thyroid works very hard to support and provide our foetus with the thyroid hormone; it almost goes into a period of hyperthyroidism. Typically, post pregnancy, if you have taken care to eat right, sleep well and exercise, the thyroid gland will bounce back to normal functioning.

But of course that's easier said than done. Newborn babies barely sleep through nights, so for a mother to sleep well is almost impossible. Post pregnancy, most young mothers are in a state of confusion about what is really good for them. She has to listen to what her mother says, mother-in-law says, the latest women's magazine says or some Pinky aunty's neighbour's daughter says, so to end the confusion she resorts to finishing that ice cream tub in the freezer. And work out? Well, one is so tired changing nappies and feeding, that workouts and gyms seem to exist on some other planet. All in all, in this situation, it's difficult to support the thyroid, but with a little awareness and planning we can do it. The hormonal shift during pregnancy and the shift in lifestyle post pregnancy make the thyroid susceptible to hypothyroidism. So plan pregnancies in advance by eating right at least a year in advance and create avenues for rest and recovery post pregnancy.

Menopause is another time when there is a huge shift in the hormonal environment. It's again a period of confusion about what exactly to expect, and we are often told that a bit of weight gain is inevitable around this phase. False again. Hormonally you are going through a phase called 'estrogen dominance', which means normal levels of estrogen and lower levels of progesterone. This does block your thyroid production a bit and there is always a chance that you may develop 'hypothyroid symptoms', though there may be no case for hypothyroidism as per blood reports. By symptoms, I mean weakness, fatigue, irritability, poor complexion, hair loss, weight gain, bloating, etc. Then of course there are lifestyle and social issues. Most women haven't learnt to speak their mind or haven't learnt to take a break. Working without a break for years together and learning to live with stress puts your thyroid at further risk. Add to that teenage children and indifferent, or worse, demanding partners, and you are clearly overworking the thyroid. So again, with menopause, one needs to equip oneself to cope with both the hormonal as well as lifestyle changes.

Trying too many diets, going to every weight-loss farm, overdoing exercise, being constantly in a state of flux — thin for two months and fat for five months — being on calorie-restricted food, taking 'fat burners' to lose weight and generally pushing yourself to do a lot more than what you have the energy for are all fertile grounds for thyroid malfunction.

What can I do about it?

Tons of things. If we understand that our problem (weight gain or weight loss because of a hypo or hyper thyroid respectively) is not because of the thyroid itself, then there are tons of things that we can or ought to do. Know that hypo or hyper thyroid conditions both overwork the thyroid gland, so look at your body beyond weight loss and don't tell yourself that I'd rather have a hyper thyroid. A malfunctioning or overworked thyroid finds it difficult to carry out all its tasks, and remember, cellular respiration or uptake of oxygen by your cells is one of them. So work at supporting your thyroid in every possible way. I have listed out the main strategies below. Whether you are hypo or hyper, the points below will help because they are aimed at supporting the thyroid function at peak efficiency so that you get to your optimum body composition and body weight.

Nutrition strategies

- First things first, improve intake of iodine. Before the government decided to iodise our salt, we (Indians) had a lot of cases of goitre. In fact, those of you who are thirty and older will remember seeing women, mostly rural, with huge necks — they almost looked like there was a ball in their necks. That was an iodine deficiency, goitre, another form of thyroid malfunction. It's not so common now, thanks to iodised salt. But it's not just iodised salt that has iodine; a lot of our natural foods that we avoid eating because we think we are fat are actually rich in iodine. Tragic isn't it? Isn't it time we think of our food in terms of the nutrients they provide, and not calories? Or would we rather be on thyroid replacement therapy (fancy name for popping t4 thyroxine/altroxine/thyronom and the like), which eventually teaches our thyroid to not produce its own t4? So come on, let's consume all the nutrients that we need to support a healthy thyroid function, and even if we are taking the morning thyroid pill, let's work at reducing the dosage and finally going drug-free.

- Some iodine-rich foods that we avoid when we go on a 'diet' are bananas, carrots, strawberries, milk and whole grains. I think you can understand why I put bananas, carrots, strawberries and milk in the list of foods we avoid — clearly because they are 'high calorie' and 'fattening'. Gosh! Besides their numerous nutrients, they've got iodine and can help pump it into your thyroid cells, and of course if you are pregnant, lactating or nearing menopause, you need it more than ever. Our thyroid plays a role in the homeostasis of calcium and glucose (it's involved in calcium absorption and glucose metabolism), which means without adequate iodine supply in your diet, you will even become vulnerable to osteoporosis and diabetes.

- Whole grains, read carbs, which is the other food group that we are asked to restrict, if not avoid, when we are on a 'weight-loss diet', are again an iodine-rich source. So please give up on your salad and soup routines and get back to eating your rice, bhakris, rotis, etc. And yes, please eat them with sabzi, because green leafy vegetables and other seasonal vegetables can provide iodine as well. And don't forget dal, dahi or kadhi as an accompaniment, because you need to complete your amino acid profile; remember tyrosine? And phenylalanine, that essential amino acid, to make tyrosine which you will get only if you have good, complete sources of protein.
- So that brings us to good complete sources of protein: cheese, paneer, whey protein, milk, curd, dals eaten with whole grains and eggs, fresh seafood and chicken if you are a non-vegetarian. Here's something funny. On one of my treks to Sikkim, the guide said to me, 'Toh aap "non-meter" ho.' What? I asked. Non-meter = no meat and meter = meat-eaters, he explained. So depending on whether you are a meter or non-meter, choose your proteins wisely. If you are a non-meter, you may need to use high-quality protein supplements like whey protein. Again, as weight-loss victims, we are asked to avoid eating good protein sources. Cheese and paneer are out for being 'fattening', and even if we are allowed dals, it's only without rice and roti, so the little protein that we do consume is incomplete and therefore useless to the body.

- In fact, while on diets, we are allowed such little food and we are on such restricted calories, that even if our thyroid is functioning perfectly normally, it starts slowing down, trying to match its metabolism to the low-calorie diet. And then of course, if we already have hypothyroidism, the diet further weakens our thyroid action by teaching it to slow down more to match the low-calorie diet.
- All in all, if you have a thyroid 'problem', you will need to eat more and you need to increase your calorie intake by consuming more wholesome meals. Got that? **Reassure and support your thyroid with the essential amino acids, good quality carbs (unprocessed), iodine, and start taking vitamins B, C and E supplements.** Increased nutrient and therefore calorie intake not just supports the thyroid, but it also reassures and encourages it to improve metabolism to match the increased intake.
- Of course, remember that the nutrient to calorie ratio is at the crux of increasing calorie intake. If you start celebrating after reading 'increase calories' and throw yourself a biscuit (however low calorie), ice cream (however fat free) and chips (whichever grain or 'oil free') party, then your thyroid will ruin your party and vice-versa. All processed foods, no matter how sugar-free or fat-free they claim they may be, are rich in salt. When you eat too much salt, then you upset the fine balance of sodium and potassium in your cells (details in Chapter 3) and make it impossible for your thyroid to absorb the iodine that's being pumped at it (now you

know why you only have juices and low-fat biscuits and still feel bloated — disturbed sodium and potassium balance). **So remember, increase calories but not at the cost of increasing salt and processed food**. Just have good old homemade and wholesome food.

Peanuts, gobi, soya

If you've got hypothyroid, you've probably been told that peanuts, gobi and soya are banned for you. Why a blanket ban? Apparently, it's not good for hypothyroid? Really, why? Most people who've authoritatively given you this information won't know why or won't have a very convincing answer. But here's the truth behind the ban. These foods can interfere with iodine absorption, but (and this is a BIG but) only if you consume them raw.

Now your peanuts are roasted, the gobi's been made into a sabzi and soya will be in the form of either milk or tofu (and chunks if you are still stupid enough to believe that they are 'protein rich'. No they're not, soy milk and tofu are far superior protein choices). Cooking these foods reduces the antagonist properties of these foods against iodine absorption. So, please, bindaas khao. I mean, just think about it, if the malice 'they' are spreading against peanuts and gobi (in fact the entire cabbage family — broccoli, cauliflower, green cabbage, red cabbage) was actually true, then what about our 'aloo-gobi population'. All of north India dabbaos gobi in the form of sabzi or gobi paratha and even gobi achar. Is there an epidemic of hypothyroidism from Delhi to Kashmir? Similarly, peanuts or groundnuts will find their way into every dish that's cooked in Konkan all the way down to the coastal belt of Karnataka: are we all suffering from the great thyroid disease? (God! And then what will happen to Lonavala chiki?)

The thyroid can't improve or deteriorate because of one thing that you will do or not do. In fact, biscuits, cakes, chocolates, alcohol are a hundred times worse for the thyroid than gobi, peanuts and soya — but are you ever warned against them? Nope! You are sold expensive 'sugar-free, low-fat' versions of these items. And they don't stop at that, they even tell you, Come on, you can't stop enjoying life, so eat stuff which wreaks havoc on your thyroid and be my client forever, dear.

Please note that peanuts and soy are good sources of protein and essential fatty acids, so don't leave them out of your diet. And the cabbage family can lend support to your efforts to eat right by providing you with good amounts of fibre, vitamin B and the microminerals too. So no blanket bans, please.

Exercise strategies

That working out or exercise is a non-negotiable aspect of life, is an essential agreement between you and me, but why is it absolutely necessary for you to exercise if you are hypothyroid? To lose weight? No. To improve delivery and uptake of oxygen by the cells, which will ultimately lead to fat loss. The state where you get mukti from constantly yo-yoing with your body weight.

- It's very crucial that you don't overdo exercise, though, because a malfunctioning thyroid is already a sign of poor recovery. Eating right, sleeping peacefully and working out in a structured manner will ensure that you reap the benefits of exercise without overburdening your already tired body.
- Cardio or stamina-building exercises are a must to improve mobility of fatty acids in your system (hypothyroid puts you at risk of increasing circulating fats like triglycerides). **Try and perform cardio exercises that will not stress your weight-bearing joints like knee, ankle, lower back and hips.** Cycling and swimming are superb options that provide a good cardio-respiratory stimuli to the heart and lungs while not stressing your joints, tendons, bones, ligaments.

- The thyroid gland secretes t4, t3 yes, but also produces another hormone called calcitonin. Calcitonin works at putting calcium back into the bones. When the thyroid function slows down, it reduces the action of calcitonin too, putting your joints, tendons, bones, ligaments at risk as well as putting you at risk of developing low vitamin D levels (though this is more common after years of exposure to artificial thyroxine).
- **Spend at least one day a week weight-training,** because when you move around with excess weight, the musculoskeletal system needs some serious strengthening to keep you injury-free. Strong muscles, tendons and ligaments protect your weight-bearing joints and provide stimuli for your bones to store more calcium, thus supporting the action of calcitonin.
- **Yoga learned from an experienced teacher can be of amazing value**. Often my clients tell me that sarvangasana is great for the thyroid. See it's like this: first of all you have to learn to perform the sarvangasana with a certain degree of effortlessness (sthiram, sukham iti asana, said Patanjali; it means for your posture to be called an asana, it needs to be steady and happy). To lift the lower body above your head and to hold it against gravity while balancing your weight on your shoulders is no mean task, and to be able to get there you have to first practise many basic poses or yogasanas like trikonasana, tadasana, etc., which are 'not popular' for the thyroid.
- There is no one pill, no one asana, no one thing that you can do for your thyroid. You must be prepared

to work on all common sense approaches to help strengthen your system, even if they are not popular for 'helping/curing' hypothyroid. Asanas learnt under expert guidance work on creating a fine balance in the system and work on every single cell of the body, so if you don't get time through the week, find yourself a weekend class. FYI, Padma Vibhushan BKS Iyengar, legend and encyclopaedia on yogasana, once famously told his students, 'In my opinion if you learn to do the tadasana (simply standing still) well, then you don't have to spend time practising any other yoga pose.' The point is, it's not about how many exotic or convoluted postures you can get into, it's about mastering the asana, and learning to steady yourself in the most basic of asanas or tasks of life.

The morning thyroid pill and mitahar

What happens to Principle 1, 'Eat within ten minutes of rising', if you have to take your thyroid pill first thing in the morning? Well, tweak that principle and make it forty minutes post taking the thyroid pill. The hormone replacement therapy that you are on (ya, I am talking about the thyroxine [t4] tab that you take) is going to interfere with micro-nutrient absorption, so take your vitamins (the multivitamin or vitamin B tablet) only after two hours of taking the thyroid pill. So all vitamins should be taken after Meal 2.

And what about the thyroid pill and early morning workouts, especially if you are short on time? The forty-sixty minute gap that you are asked to keep between taking the thyroid pill and eating something cuts into your crucial morning hours, especially your workout time. Reaching the gym on an empty stomach is not just a guarantee for poor exercise performance but also injuries like sprains, strains, muscle pulls, etc. So then what? Speak to your doctor. Most doctors will be happy to work out an alternative time for you when you are on a relatively empty stomach (because the t4 interferes with nutrient absorption and gets absorbed better when you are on an empty stomach). So you can wake up and eat according to the first principle, hit the gym, work out, have a hearty breakfast and go about your day. Your regular workouts will help your thyroid function better and all that you will need to do is stick to taking the pill at that alternative timing that's been worked out for you. Good deal?

Sleep strategies

Let me say this one more time, **hypothyroid is a sign of poor recovery, so sleeping well and waking up fresh are the cornerstones of supporting the thyroid function.** One of the characteristics of an unsupported hypothyroid is feeling sluggish and sleepy through the day and an inability to sleep peacefully at night. (Remember the example of the lady in Chapter 1, with whom all I felt like doing was letting her sleep? Well she did have hypothyroid, and yes, on our third meeting, I did dim the lights and walked out of my office, and she slept uninterrupted for a full twenty minutes.) We all need a good night's sleep. And we all know how zombie-like we feel and yuck we look on mornings when we have twisted, turned too much in the bed and raided the fridge at night. When we sleep well, both the mind and body get a chance to restore a sense of balance and peace, crucial for every cell, hormone, enzyme, organ, tendon, muscle, bone, joint, nerve, etc. in our bodies.

IGF-I or 'Insulin-like Growth Factor' is another hormone that gets secreted by our body when it falls into restorative sleep. This hormone is responsible for a person's ability to recover and grow and allows our cells to absorb nutrients that they need once they are in the blood stream. So to support the thyroid, we need good levels of IGF-I, a) to allow our thyroid cells to absorb the nutrients it needs, and b) to protect us from developing insulin insensitivity or diabetes.

Sleep is also crucial because hypothyroid is affected by what is now being called as 'adrenal fatigue'. Cortisol, commonly called the 'stress hormone', is secreted when the adrenal gland learns to perpetually stay in the 'flight or fight' mode. Hypothyroidism is eventually a condition caused by either hormonal or lifestyle stress, or a combination of both, so expect your adrenals to feel the fatigue. Create good conditions for sleep, and sleep fearlessly in the afternoon for about thirty minutes.

Also, without good sleep, you get zero results out of exercise. So if you plan to seriously exercise, learn to sleep well first. And eating right is a good place to start. It creates the right environment in the body for a restful and not drugged sleep.

And here's a pointer: if you can, then don't wake yourself up every morning with an irritating alarm; instead allow the body to wake up naturally. It's a sign of a good sleep and excellent recovery.

Relationship strategies

Ah! Yes, they affect our thyroid too, simply because our relationships — or lack of them — affect our overall health. It's important to invest time in cultivating and maintaining meaningful relationships, especially with people that we interact with regularly. Having said that, the most important part of the relationship strategy to reduce the load on an overworked thyroid, is the ability to say 'NO'. Say it with me — N.O., NO! Women who haven't developed the skill to say NO are the ones who usually haven't developed an understanding of what to expect out of themselves. On the one hand, they are expert givers — to children, family, friends, colleagues, domestic staff, etc., everybody's fall-back option. On the other hand, they are always left wanting — of others understanding that they are too tired right now, or must they just do this on their own? But hey, who the f*&$ is asking us to run ourselves ragged keeping up with demanding relationships — mother-in-law wants to shop/maths homework with daughter/movie with husband/presentation at work/making aachar at mom's/babysitting friend's kid, etc. In every language, there is a word for NO, just learn to say it. And seriously, get over yourself. Just because you didn't do it doesn't mean things don't or won't get done. They will, give it a try, and in case they really don't get done, you already have the expertise and super speciality skill of getting things back on track, right? I am guessing you have realised by this time that you get no medal, trip to Switzerland, gourmet dinner at doorstep, acknowledgement certificate or much less appreciation for being there for everybody every single time, so learn to be there for yourself once in a while. Say no, learn to excuse yourself from all the assumed tasks and responsibilities and listen to your inner voice.

According to the tantric philosophy (and all the eastern sciences and philosophies), the thyroid is considered the sacred voice and corresponds to the throat chakra. A malfunctioning thyroid usually means that you are so busy with life that you haven't found the time or space to hear yourself. Remember how Nandini (Chapter 1) took calls from her daughter, slogged at work, confirmed a date with her husband — all small things, but having an accumulative effect on her stress and TSH levels, ultimately overworking her thyroid. The fact that we haven't learnt to reassert ourselves or talk about our innermost feelings to people who really matter, also adds to the burden. To support our thyroid, we must learn to speak our mind, tactfully yes, but speak for sure. It's often said that women the world over speak the language of silence, and in that process harm themselves and society at large. A lot of women's rights issues are really all about women keeping silent over concerns that need to be made a big noise about or discussed openly and compassionately at public forums.

Alright, I guess I am digressing but here's the long and short of the relationship strategy: learn to say NO and make time to listen to your inner voice (I mean come on, listening to her inner voice Sonia Gandhi gave up the post of prime minister and made Dr Manmohan Singh prime minister. Worked well for us, right?). Here's an idea, take a break (plan for it in advance, of course) for three-four days every three-four months and spend time chilling. Howzzaat? Say that it's therapy for your thyroid. ☺

The Dalai Lama once tweeted: To know what you have done in the past look at your body, to know what you will do in the future look at your mind. And here's my addition, chote muh badi baat (forgive me Dalai Lamaji) — to look at what you are currently doing, look at your thyroid.

The thyroid pill

So if the problem is not an isolated 'thyroid problem', as we have learnt it never is, just taking a pill is not going to resolve it. In most hypothyroid cases, you will simply be asked to take some form or other of t4, but that hardly ever solves the problem, and that's exactly why you will see other women around you taking the drug forever and ever and still having a 'thyroid problem'. The thyroid is only manifesting the problem, not creating it.

If you are already on the early morning pill, then read the strategies that much more carefully, because you need to support your thyroid function more than ever. And don't live in the hope that popping a pill will help you lose weight or complain that even after taking the thyroid medicine you haven't lost weight. I am guessing you have understood by now that just popping a pill is not going to help; lifestyle changes will.

Patronise doctors who believe strongly in lifestyle changes like eating right, working out regularly, sleeping on time and having meaningful relationships whether at home or work. Also doctors who understand that a lack of these factors exposes you to more conditions than ever, and are willing to actively encourage you to change your lifestyle over simply scribbling prescriptions and at the most saying, 'You must lose weight' or 'Go for a walk' or 'Start exercising', while they are scribbling. Mere lip service to lifestyle changes given without eye contact.

Typically, doctors who invest time in working out, eating right and regularising sleeping hours are the ones who have a strong belief in making lifestyle changes to overcome or control (depending on when you catch it) diseases. They believe in them because they have reaped the benefits themselves and are constantly in touch with friends/acquaintances/patients who have reaped the many rewards. They are fearless about weaning you off dosages, and are happy to walk you to a drug-free state. They also understand enough about drugs to know that the drug can cause side-effects or conditions as dangerous as the disease itself, if not more. Also work with doctors who invest in updating themselves regularly, at least once a year, or those who take study breaks (it's a sign of a responsible doctor, somebody who is willing to let go of his/her daily [big fat] earning to slog it out in school or courses). The rate at which medical science is progressing, it makes sense to stay in touch with the latest, and now of course medical science, especially allopathy (ayurveda, homeopathy, unani and other traditional medical practices have always believed in it), is waking up to the fact that lifestyle changes are crucial for defeating diseases, or at least to ensure optimum or maximum action of prescription drugs and to reduce their side-effects.

How will I know that I am getting better?

Once you wake up fresh, sleep soundly, feel strong in your bones and joints, see an improvement in your stamina and your skin feels better, you should know that the thyroid is feeling supported and will bounce back to peak efficiency functioning. You simply must keep at practising lifestyle changes day in and day out. An improvement in overall health is often associated with an improvement in body composition (more weight of muscle and bone, less weight of fat tissue) and does eventually lead to weight loss. But the reverse — lose weight and you will feel better — is not true. Everything depends on what you lost — bone, muscle or fat. And also what you gained.

Real life diet analysis

Sneha Kulkarni is a sixty-six-year-old TV artiste and a homemaker.

She has been suffering from thyroid, diabetes and high blood pressure for the past three-four years. She also has knee pain and digestion problems (stomach gets bloated and has constipation).

She has long days and is constantly busy with household responsibilities, her own work and taking care of her seventy-five-year-old ailing husband.

In her attempt to portray herself as the 'ideal' wife, she has compromised on many things, including her style of cooking and eating (basically given up her favourite foods). She has adapted to her husband's taste in food (they are from different regions and had different styles of food preparation). In fact, she thinks her cooking style, which uses peanuts and coconut, is tasty but unhealthy.

She is concerned about her health and therefore tries to eat 'healthy' (Herbalife milkshakes, Splenda instead of sugar, was her concept of healthy) and has also been to various dieticians in the past. She has gone for days surviving on veggie juices, salads, black tea and pani puri water (this logic beats me)!

Sneha had a lot of responsibilities including work and an ailing husband, and the additional stress of crash dieting amidst all this only led her to a state of depression.

But Sneha was brave enough to opt for immediate treatment to help her out of that miserable state.

Three-day diet recall

Time	Food/Drink	Activity Recall	Workout
Day 1			
5.30 a.m.		Woke up	
5.50 a.m.		Got ready for Hasya club	
5.50 a.m.	1 pear		
6.20 a.m.		Drove 1 km to Hasya club	
6.30 – 7.30 a.m.		Yoga	Pranayam and Hasya yoga
7.45 a.m.	1 peda (clubs are full of these)		
7.45 a.m.		Got back home, went up by lift	
8.15 – 8.30 a.m.	2 dosas with chutney + 1 cup tea with Splenda		
8.30 – 9 a.m.		Read newspaper, made calls	
9 – 9.30 a.m.		Gupshup with my bai	
9.30 a.m.		Bathed	
10.00 a.m.		Went to flat on lower floor to meet husband	
10.15 a.m.	Herbalife milkshake		
10.45 a.m.		Was driven to dentist for treatment of abscess and to fix canine	
12.15 p.m.		Returned home	
12.30 p.m.	Had 2 glasses of water		
1.20 p.m.	¾ bhakri, 2 tsp pithale, 1 serving spoon cooked rice, 1 katori mango pickle		

3.30 p.m.	1 cup tea + 2 pieces chakli + 2 glasses water		
5.00 p.m.	1 mango (small)		
7.35 p.m.	1 glass milkshake (Herbalife)		
7 – 9 p.m.		Watched TV	
9 p.m.	1 mid-sized bowl oats khichdi + 1 katori moong dal varan + mango pickle + ½ katori matar usal + 1 tbsp pithale + 2 tbsp kakdi raita		
9.30 – 10.15 p.m.		Cleared table and washed dishes	
10.15 p.m.		Went to bed	
Day 2			
5.30 a.m.		Woke up	
5.45 a.m.	1 pear		
5.45 – 6.15 a.m.		Got ready for Hasya club	
6.15 a.m.		Drove 1 km to the club	
6.20 – 7.30 a.m.			Practised yoga
7.30 – 8.10 a.m.		Gupshup	
8.15 a.m.		Drove back home	
8.20 – 8.30 a.m.	Two slices bread with 1 cheese slice toasted + 1 cup tea with Splenda		
8.30 – 9.00 a.m.		Made and received phone calls	
9.15 a.m.		Bathed	
9.30 - 9.45 a.m.		Gupshup with my bai	

9.45 – 10.15 a.m.		Internet banking	
10.15 a.m.		Downstairs to meet husband	
10.15 – 11.15 a.m.	1 cup coffee + toast	Gupshup with my husband	
11.15 – 11.25 a.m.		Put room in order	
11.25 a.m. – 1 p.m.		Discussed a teaching assignment with friends	
1.15 – 1.35 p.m.	2 polis + 1 katori moong dal waran + matar cauliflower bhaji		
1.40 – 2.15 p.m.		Napped	
2.30 p.m.	½ glass Herbalife milkshake		
2.45 p.m.		Was driven to Mahindra Resorts office	
5.15 p.m.	1 cup tea + Splenda + 2 slices of toast + 2 glasses water		
Till 5.40 p.m.		Reorganised Mahindra file	
5.40 – 6.40 p.m.			Went for a walk
7.15 p.m.	Herbalife milkshake - 1 glass		
7 – 9 p.m.		Watched TV	
9 p.m.	1 bhakri + vagyanchi bhaji - 2 servings + chavli palak bhaji + 1 vati moong dal waran		
9.30 – 10.15 p.m.		Cleared table and washed vessels	
10.15 p.m.		Went to bed	

Day 3 (Holiday)			
6 a.m.		Woke up	
6.30 a.m.	1 apple + 1 glass water		
7.30 a.m.		Bathed and got ready for a function	
8.30 a.m.	Tea + sugar + 2 slices mava cake		
9.30 a.m.	4 idlis + chutney + 1 serving rava sheera		
10.15 a.m.		Took a small walk and participated in the thread ceremony	
12.00 p.m.	1 cup tea + 1 slice mava cake	Gupshup with relatives till 1.30 p.m.	
1.30 p.m.	Masala bhaat + turaichya dal waran + 2 servings mixed veg + beans usal + 2 small glasses matha + ¾ katori basundi		
3 p.m.		Drove down back to Pune (driver)	
4 p.m.	2 cups tea + 2 slices mava cake		
5.30 – 6.30 p.m.			Went for a walk
7 p.m.	1 glass milk		
9 p.m.	1 katori moong + waran + 1 serving palak bhaji + 1½ bhakri		
9.30 – 10 p.m.		Cleared table and washed up dishes	
10.00 p.m.		Went to bed	

Evaluation of the recall

Sneha has been a victim of crash dieting in her hope to lose weight and remain slim (read: not healthy) for life.

She was already suffering from a thyroid malfunction, diabetes, blood pressure, all of which are lifestyle disorders arising due to stress, wrong eating habits, lack of exercise and nutrient deprivation.

Crash diets put the body under tremendous stress. Whenever the body is under stress, it releases stress hormones (cortisol) that in turn lead to a hormonal imbalance in your body and increase your nutrient requirements. Along with the release of stress hormones, the body's lean body mass — muscle mass and bone mineral density — is also compromised on (which in Sneha's case lead to knee and bone problems).

So the crash dieting actually aggravated her health condition instead of resolving it. Because of her thyroid condition, she needed to provide her body with wholesome foods along with regular exercise to improve her hormonal functioning. Instead, she was depriving herself of good healthy food.

Modifications

Sneha simply needed to make the right food choices and eat well- balanced meals and also eat to satisfy her taste buds. She mainly needed to create a stress-free environment in her body so that it would be able to maximise the absorption of nutrients. (Whenever the body is mentally or physically stressed, absorption is very poor.)

She also needed to exercise regularly (weight-training particularly) to improve her lean body mass. Regular exercise helps in reducing stress, improves the immune system function, and also improves metabolism. Thus it will help in improving the thyroid hormone function and the cells also become more sensitised to hormonal action. Weight-training will also improve her bone mineral density as it helps the bones retain calcium.

She also joined a 'Hasya club' where she met like-minded people. They took up breathing and stretching exercises as well in this club, which helped her unwind and relax. (A calm state of mind also helps balance hormones.)

She can modify her diet as follows:

Meal 1 (5.45 a.m.): Banana

Meal 2 (7.30 a.m.): Poha/upma/idli

Meal 3 (9.30 a.m.): Handful of peanuts

Meal 4 (11.30 a.m.): Glass of buttermilk

Meal 5 (12.30 p.m.): Rice + dal + bhaji or khichdi + veg

Meal 6 (2.30 p.m.): 2 egg whites

Meal 7 (4.30 p.m.): Vegetable toast

Meal 8 (6.30 p.m.): Whey protein shake

Meal 9 (8.00 p.m.): Fish/chicken + rice + sabzi

She was also advised to take calcium and vitamin D supplements in order to improve her bone mineral density and thyroid functioning. Vitamin B-complex (B6, B12), Omega-3, selenium, zinc, amino acids (whey protein) were also introduced, which together would contribute to improving thyroid hormone sensitivity and functioning.

Sneha adapted to all these lifestyle changes very comfortably. She also followed her diet to the T, except for a few slip-ups on certain days. She was also regular with her exercise.

She started enjoying her food and because of this her nutrient absorption and assimilation also improved. After forty years of marriage, she started cooking according to her traditional style and genes, bringing back coconut and peanuts as part of her diet. Not only did this satisfy her taste buds, but coconut and peanut — which contain essential fats — actually helped lubricate her bones and joints, which relieved her knee pain.

She was motivated enough to feel responsible for herself and not just for her husband. She had started looking at herself with much more affection and this greatly helped her improve her overall health and understanding towards her body.

As a result of all these changes, she started feeling more energetic, and she was able to take care of her husband without stressing about it. As her well-being improved, her husband's health also started improving ☺.

Within two months of making all these changes, her thyroid hormone functioning had improved. With gradual reduction in the dosage, she has now been completely weaned off the medication.

She has now adapted to these changes as a way of life and feels that she has never before enjoyed such great fitness levels while being on a 'diet'.

3

PCOD/PCOS

What is it?

Whatever it is, it seems to be spreading like an epidemic and is fast becoming everybody's favourite condition to blame their weight gain on! So before we go further into figuring out whether we should blame weight gain or an inability to lose weight on this 'curse', let's get its name right. PCOD — polycystic ovary (or ovarian) disease and PCOS — polycystic ovary (or ovarian) syndrome are like same-same but different. PCOD means that your ovaries are reeling under pressure and feeling the brunt of the disturbances in your body and generally not functioning at their peak efficiency. PCOS means that these disturbances are now no longer just in the ovaries but are also manifesting in other parts of the body — as acne and body hair to put the mildest first. 'Syndrome' is actually like a set or 'package' of symptoms that you get with the 'curse': irregular periods, obesity, insulin insensitivity, high amounts of 'male hormones', irritability, high blood pressure, difficulty in conceiving, oily skin, thinning hair, to name a few.

Now the main problem with this curse is that it often gets 'diagnosed' and 'treated' only after you have been 'trying' to get pregnant for a while. Typically, women who have been married for a while and are having regular intercourse without contraceptives but failing to conceive will be taken to a doctor and declared to have PCOS. Now because the terms PCOD and PCOS are often used for each other, I will use the term PCOS (because I like how it sounds and hear it the most), but know that whether you have PCOD, PCOS or PCO (the last is characterised by the presence of small cysts around the surface of the ovaries; not all women who have PCO have PCOD/ PCOS), everything in here will be helpful for you. In fact, the following information will also be helpful to you if you have a thick endometrium and high prolactin.

Before we delve into the realms of our hormones, there are some things that I would like to put down:

- Our body and mind, more specifically, their well-being (or lack of it) affects our hormones.
- Our hormones, in turn, affect the well-being of our mind and body.
- Since PCOS is a hormonal condition, you are up against a vicious cycle and it is normal to feel frustrated.
- Having said that, being frustrated doesn't help. (It may earn you a label though, 'frustu' or 'full frustu', depending on how generous people around you are.)
- There is a saying, 'Complain or do something about it'. Taking inspiration from it, I've coined my own: **'To break out of a vicious cycle, start working with the known factors to control the unknown.'**
- (Thanks for the applause for my creativity; let's get to the point.) Between hormones and the body, we know the body better since we can see, touch, feel it every day.

- So let's start working with our body to influence the 'unknown', i.e. our hormones, to which we have little or almost no direct access (mostly we 'feel' hormones only through changes in our body).
- Nobody knows the exact cause of PCOS; it is largely agreed, though, that dropping body fat (that's exactly what your doctor meant when he/she said 'you need to lose some weight') helps the ovaries function better and therefore overcome PCOS.
- On this premise I shall say (no marks for guessing) that I am sceptical about conventional ways of 'treating' PCOS: contraceptives (Yasmin/Diane and the likes) with or without an anti-diabetic drug (metmorfin/Glucophage, etc.) and with or without a diuretic or anti-androgen drugs (Aldactone, etc.).
- Overriding the ovaries or trying to bring about a 'hormonal balance' by using golis has many issues, not the least of which is the side effects of these drugs. FYI, in Mumbaiya we say, 'Goli mat de', which means 'Stop fooling around'.
- It also means we are trying to work with the unknown to influence the known.
- The more you try grappling with the unknown, the more lost (and fat) you feel.
- So everything that you will read below is the way to use what is within your control (your body) to influence the unknown, which seems to be going out of your control.

Coming back to where we started, the main 'problem' with PCOS is not the fear that it may prevent you from getting and staying pregnant, but the fact that it's stressing your ovaries and affecting the delicate hormonal balance our body tries to keep, day in and day out, minute by minute. Basically, makes it tiresome for your body to maintain good health and immune functions.

Alright girls, we basically need to support our ovaries, and to be able to support our ovaries we need to know a bit about them.

Where are your ovaries? (Before that, ovary is singular and ovaries is plural and since we have two of them, like eyes and ears, we tend to call them ovaries. And mind you, if you don't mind *them,* well then they start rhyming with worries. Ovaries — worries, ovary — worry. Get it?) So ovaries are in the lower part of our abdomen, in the pelvic region, above our vagina. We go about our lives, doing god knows what, and then we stand in front of the mirror and say, 'Yeh mera lower stomach, yeh jana chahiye,' or 'Everything else is okay but my lower abs are bulging out'. Boss, all that fat is sitting right on top of your ovaries, suffocating them, making it difficult for them to breathe, so please, your kind attention is solicited.

Hormonally vibrant

As women, we are what I call 'hormonally vibrant'. We get easily bored with one kind of hormone dominating our system, and since we believe in democracy and equal opportunity, we allow our ovaries to be influenced by different hormones every few days. They (the hormones) in turn, if we allow them full freedom of expression, help us to keep our ovaries strong, well-nourished, oxygenated and vibrant. Ovaries affect the health of our body, and the health of our body affects the vibrancy of our ovaries. Since we're working on the premise that we can influence our body much more easily than our hormones, we will keep talking about what we need to do with our body to make our ovaries healthy. This rhythmic rise and fall of hormones that happens in our ovaries, almost like a well-choreographed sequence, expresses itself as 'periods' or 'chums' or menses in our body. Of course we know that this is not just a four, five or seven-day event. When you watch a one-hour breathtaking choreographed dance on stage, performed effortlessly by nubile dancers, we know that they must have practised, practised, practised for hours, days and who knows even months together to put up this one-hour show.

Similarly, for our periods to come effortlessly (regularly), without cramps, mood-swings, etc. our hormones, like the dancers, must work patiently, dedicatedly and practise their moves to perfection under the guidance of a masterji (choreographer). Let's think of hormones as the dancers, rising and falling, twirling and moving; the ovary as the rehearsal stage; the anterior pituitary (you know her right? read the previous chapter?) as the masterji; the hypothalamus (you know her too) as the organiser of the show and the body as the main platform where the grand event called menses will be performed. You're still with me, right? Okay, so let's look at what's happening behind the scenes of this spectacular event called menses or periods:

Main event: Menses Day 0 – Day 5	Estrogen and progesterone levels drop low Hypothalamus secretes GnRH* to stimulate the pituitary Pituitary releases LH** and FSH♦ (typically more FSH than LH) slowly and steadily	LH and FSH start producing several follicles (3-30) in the ovary Follicle is like a swelling around the egg (blister type) Follicles starts producing estrogen
Follicular phase Day 6 – Day 14	The dominant (primary) follicles secrete max estrogen and keep growing bigger Estrogen levels in the blood start rising LH and FSH stay low and steady, supporting the follicle to reach maturity	The uterine lining grows due to estrogen stimulation The cervix lining is thin and watery The dominant follicle is ready with mature egg
Ovulatory phase Day 15 Max chances of fertilisation of egg (chances of fertilisation go up if sperm is already present in the system or reproductive tract)	High estrogen levels signal the brain that it's time for ovulation Hypothalamus secretes massive amounts of GnRH Pituitary responds with LH and FSH surge (more LH than FSH) The mid-cycle LH/FSH peak lasts for about twenty-four hours	The pressure inside the follicle goes up and an enzymatic action breaks open the follicle releasing the mature egg The mature egg travels to the fallopian tubes (can survive max 12 to 24 hours) Remainder of follicle (corpus luteum) stays in the ovary Corpus luteum secretes progesterone and estrogen Uterus lining is at its thickest, full of nutrients and well hydrated, ready to receive the egg Cervix mucus at its thinnest
Luteal phase Day 16 – Day 28	LH and FSH levels drop to low and steady levels Estrogen levels begin to drop but get pushed up by the production of progesterone and estrogen by the corpus luteum	The egg starts moving through the tube aided by hair-like projections Uterine lining stays thick to welcome the egg Progesterone levels thicken the mucus of the cervix to stop entry of sperm or bacteria

If fertilisation occurs, embryo secretes another gonadotropin, HCG••	HCG stimulates corpus luteum to produce estrogen and progesterone	Pregnant, and you skip your period
If there is no fertilisation	The corpus luteum starts shrinking and dying Estrogen and progesterone levels drop	The egg passes out of the uterus. Uterine lining shed Menses starts Take it from the top☺

*Gonadotropin-releasing hormone
**Leutenising hormone
• Follicle stimulating hormone
•• Human chorionic gonadotropin

The story of our ovaries

Okay, I agree it's a bit technical. But here's the story in words:

The show organiser (hypothalamus) thinks boss, ek grand event karna chahiye. She has the money (gonadotropin-releasing hormone, GnRH) but not the skill to teach dancing or to spot talent. So she employs a well-known choreographer (pituitary) for the job. On receiving money (GnRH), pituitary sends her team, two teaching assistants, the hormones FSH and LH, for the job. They start talent-spotting and auditioning a dozen or more dancers (follicles which secrete estrogen).

They start putting the dancers through basic but consistent training and soon enough one of the dancers (dominant follicle) shows maximum receptiveness and potential to become the lead dancer. The lead dancer is now almost ready to show off her moves. All this practice, grooming, training is happening in the ovary, the rehearsal stage or dance studio. *The follicular stage.*

The show organiser is happy with the training and gives out some more money (GnRH) to the pituitary, who in turn puts the lead dancer through rigorous training (mid-cycle LH – FSH surge) and arranges for the grand rehearsal with costumes, make-up, etc. all in place (uterus thick to receive the egg). The grand rehearsal is thrown open to an audience too (cervix thins to allow sperms). The lead dancer puts up a great show and loses herself (follicle ruptures and releases the egg) in the performance. *The ovulation phase.*

The organiser is satisfied with the grand rehearsal and keeps the money going steady to pituitary. Pituitary's team also keeps up with regular training of the dancer (corpus luteum) and continues grooming it (producing estrogen and progesterone). *The luteal phase.*

As the main performance approaches, the dance teachers decide to taper down practice and allow the dancers to rest a bit (low levels of estrogen and progesterone).

The dancers put up a great show on the big platform that has been provided. The body experiences a beautiful, peaceful and effortless period. Alright hypothalamus, pituitary, ovary, take a bow. Good job! *Menses.*

Pregnancy is a bit like kahani mein twist. Think of it as if some scout (sperm) attends the grand rehearsal, is smitten by the main dancer who lost herself in the performance (mature egg), and asks the masterji to put her through a further nine-month training to put up an even grander show than what was initially planned. Now, not just the masterji but even the dancer herself can start practising on her own (releases HCG) which helps her growth. Nine months later, the dancer surpasses herself and puts up a brilliant show (baby is born).

The story hopefully makes it easier for us to understand menstruation and how the ovaries work under the influence of our hormones and how the hormones that our ovaries produce influence our menstruation and how that influences our body. The reality is, the enzymes which cause the follicles to rupture are all protein-based, made up of as many as a hundred amino acids. The uterine lining, which gets thicker during the cycle, needs an adequate supply of multiple nutrients — good quality carbs, essential fats, minerals, vitamins, etc. — to welcome the egg. As with all fields, the better the platform you provide, the better the performance gets. It means that more and more talent will mature and be eager to perform. Providing a good platform or body is our responsibility. The body is 'annamaya kosha', which means that it's affected by food. So if you are keen on providing a good platform to your dancers and want this delicate balance to not topple, please eat right and stop avoiding nutrients under the pretext of losing weight.

So the story above is that of regular periods. Let me take a bow for my choice of words: *regular,* not *monthly.* Because nature doesn't follow standardisation, it prefers the twenty-eight day period to stay in textbooks (mostly so that we can simplify things), but in reality it may express itself every twenty-five, thirty, who knows, forty days. The phase where it varies the most is the follicular phase, the phase where the teachers are spotting and grooming talent. Typically, the older we get and closer we get to menopause, the shorter it gets (maybe the teachers gain experience in spotting, training dancers). The luteal phase tends to stay close to fourteen days. So every woman has her own unique cycle influenced by her heredity, place of birth, weather, nutrient status, exercise status, state of mind, etc. Also the same woman can have a varied cycle every month in different phases (or even months) of her life. So this, 'Oh, my periods are delayed by two days or one week', is really an insight into how little we understand our ovaries. Of course, if you are not getting your period at all or are getting it three-four times a month, then it's a cause for worry, and you could be experiencing the classical symptom of PCOS called amenorrhea (where periods have stopped altogether) or oligomenorrhea (irregular period), the basis of which is anovulation (opposite of ovulation). It simply means that the dance teachers are grooming and training many dancers (follicles) but not even one of them is growing to full maturity, so you have no lead dancer but a lot of mediocre or average dancers not capable of being the lead (producing an egg). This forms the basis of PCOS — poly (many), cystic (follicles, growing like blisters with fluid inside them), ovarian (inside the ovary) symptom.

As I have already said, nobody knows the exact reason or cause behind this 'lot of average dancers and not even one capable of becoming the lead' issue, but there is a huge link with the lack of a good platform (unhealthy body composition or obesity) to this problem. And again, after a problem has persisted for a long time, you kind of don't know what happened first: mediocrity that led to a bad platform or a bad platform that led to mediocrity. So if high body fat made you susceptible to PCOS or PCOS led to high body fat levels, nobody knows, but we all know for sure that they influence each other. Body fat is hormonally active (it's otherwise a 'nonworking tissue' though), increasing the estrogen in your body and therefore putting other hormones off balance.

Also PCOS can occur if the teachers LH and FSH don't divide work equally between them. In PCOS, the FSH and LH ratios — which are otherwise 1:1 — tend to go for a toss, typically more LH than FSH. More LH means that there could be more than the required production of testosterone (often called the male hormone), which again affects estrogen production. The ovaries produce 'androgens' (group of male hormones) which produce testosterone. So consider androgen as a sidekick to the main dancer. No, I don't mean to run it down, only trying to explain that we need androgens like testosterone, but in the right proportion. I mean, what is Munna bhai without Circuit? But if Circuit's role is increased or decreased dramatically, then there is no fun in watching Munna bhai. Get my point? We need testosterone (to keep bone and muscle density, sex drive, etc.), but in the right proportion. As testosterone and other androgens increase, you see their effects on the 'platform', i.e. body — increase in facial hair, hair on chest, stomach, under the chin, change in body fat distribution (bigger deposits on and above the waist, smaller hips), acne, thinning hair, irritability, sometimes even depression. As the platform gets compromised, so does the teaching (LH and FSH), organiser, the money (GnRH) and talent (estrogen and progesterone). As hormones start spiralling out of balance, you start experiencing tender boobs, high body fat levels, irregular periods, heavy bleeding, insulin insensitivity, acne, hair on face, hair off the scalp, difficulty in conceiving, etc. (ya, the package). All in all, full-blown chaos.

What does it expose me to?

Well, Type 2 diabetes for one. Long-term effects include high blood pressure, leading to heart diseases, high body fat taking a toll on bones and joints, depression and, not to forget, difficulty in conceiving. The main issue with this is that there is always a chance that you don't get help till you find it difficult to get pregnant. But again, one must remember that 'getting pregnant' is not the be-all and end-all of a woman's life. Know that periods have to be regular and painless; if that's not the case with you, then you need to support your ovaries better and not silence them with a painkiller. Our 'shyness' and stupidity about discussing and understanding our menses can land us with more than one problem. As for getting pregnant, take heart that you are in India. We have technology and doctors who will even make a dining table deliver if they put their minds to it. So seriously, it's not about whether you will get pregnant, it's about how *effortlessly* you want to get pregnant. I mean think about it, more and more women seem to be suffering from PCOS, but has that brought our population down? No, instead we have them giving birth to twins and triplets.

What exposes me to this curse?

Like all curses, there is a genetic predisposition, which means if it runs in your family, you are likely to have it. Before you blame your family, know that a lot of us have this curse today without any genetic link, suggesting a strong connection to a 'modern' lifestyle instead. Lifestyle issue it surely is; I also suspect it's kind of a social issue. Look at the way our lives have changed. Women have made inroads, and successfully at that, in a 'man's world' — they are executives, managers, heads of businesses, leading teams of men and women to make tons of money, travelling more than ever, etc., so they are going beyond 'traditional' professions of teaching, cooking, designing, etc. (men are making inroads here and successfully). Basically, it's leaving women with very little time and ironically limited resources to eat (and cook) wholesome food, so the consumption of processed, quick meals (fast food) is going through the roof. This 'Had coffee for breakfast, grabbed lunch, went crazy with hunger in the evening, only reached home by 9 p.m., so the earliest dinner could be was 9.30 to 10 p.m., had a dessert post dinner' lifestyle is not a good platform to allow our one follicle (come on, it's just one; can't we support that much) to mature. Instead it's a good platform for what is called as 'insulin resistance', which shows a strong link to PCOS. Then there is the fast disappearance of open spaces, limited exercise options, crammed traffic conditions which make walking impossible and turn your fifteen-minute drive to an hour-long one — so, again inactivity and sitting in one place, which only increases your total body fat percentage and makes your weight go up as you go from school to college and from college to work.

According to me, there are 'events' which increase one's susceptibility to PCOS. These are:

- The 10th/12th Std exams where you sit long hours and especially through the nights, where you give up on that one-hour swimming class or whatever little exercise routine you had, to 'study'. You eat chips, sweets, instant noodles, etc. in the night and drink coffee, tea and, of late, 'energy drinks' to study. It's not unusual for girls to gain five to ten kilos in this phase.
- Hostel food, if you went out to study, or the fact that you spend all your pocket money on 'coffee shops and fast food' even if you live at home. Exercise? No. You are in college now, you can't run around in your compound anymore and all gyms/workout places are too far off or too expensive.
- Staying away from home to work. So you may have your own apartment or share it with roomies, but what you don't have is a functional kitchen. So office canteen and instant pizza it is.
- Shaadi-byaah. Now I wrote an entire chapter on this in *Women & the Weight Loss Tamasha*, so I won't go into details, but yeah, it increases the risk too.

The main challenge here is that we are increasingly living in situations where eating wholesome food in peace and exercising is a distant dream, but where the pressures to look thin are more than ever. Enter crash diets that further cut down on nutrients, instil a fear of food in our minds and deprive nutrients to our already overworked ovaries. Anorexia, bulimia — basically all eating disorders — lead to amenorrhea or oligomenorrhea, again not good if you want to avoid PCOS.

Eventually you have a brilliant chance to look lean, thin, sexy, whatever your buzzword is, and I am talking of forever, not just for the next big wedding/party/holiday, etc. only if your ovaries are healthy and only if we ovulate regularly.

FYI, women who don't ovulate regularly don't tend to buy sexy, fashionable or nice clothes. They'd rather hide their bodies than celebrate their womanhood. (Nice or sexy doesn't mean short and skimpy; it simply means clothes that make you feel good, attractive.)

Plastic and hormones

Our way of life has changed — we now have more plastic in our kitchen and more pesticides in our food compared to, let's say, just ten years ago. Picture your grandmom's kitchen, your mom's and then yours: how much more plastic is being used now? Now picture size, stress, health issues: you probably score more on every front.

The innumerable pesticides and fertilisers that we are now using is changing our body chemistry like never before. I don't bat an eyelid now when a fourteen-year-old emails me regarding her PCOD, or an eight-year-old turns up with diabetes (Type 2, the adult variety of diabetes). The chemicals in pesticides are making inroads all the way to our ovarian fluid and are busy penetrating deeper into our tissues. The plastic in which you carry your food, reheat, transport vegetables in and stuff take-away in, further brings chemicals into your immediate environment.

There is now a class of chemicals identified as xenoestrogen that are structurally similar to the estrogen that our body makes. The xenoestrogens are environmental polluters (air, food, water) and are a result of increased chemical use in daily life: pesticides, fertilisers, plastic, even fabric softeners, bleaching agents, mosquito and pest repellents, make-up, soaps ... the list is endless. You should worry because 'structurally similar' to our estrogen means that it will take its place in our body. It's like the gold earring you bought where you can fit different coloured drops according to the colour of your dress, or the watch whose strap you can change. Though this means more style in fashion, in our body it spells doom. When the chemical estrogen fits itself into our body, instead of the natural one we produced, it disturbs every other hormone, more specifically our androgens like testosterone. Now you know what that can mean for your ovaries: painful periods, frequent miscarriages, more cysts, high blood pressure, mood swings, more body fat... the list is endless again.

There is no easy way out. Work actively at reducing your chemical exposure. Do you really need to soften every fabric, switch on the repellent every night, reheat in plastic containers, condition your hair as many times, wash your car with detergent daily? And then do some corrective action: involve yourself in growing at least one tree, reduce garbage in your neighbourhood (to keep pests and mosquitoes out), farm your own food, go makeup free for a day every week and carry food in stainless steel containers (or at least reheat your food in glass: preferably don't reheat at all, just eat and live fresh — top to bottom, all the way).

What can I do about it?

Gosh! Tons and tons of things. Before we go further, know that effortless and regular periods are a natural consequence of optimum body fat, health and fitness levels (it means all hormones, enzymes, neurotransmitters, organs like ovaries, kidneys, liver, etc. are keeping good health). Feeling comfortable during and before periods is NORMAL. **Feeling uncomfortable, irritable, cramping during, before or after periods is ABNORMAL**. It means your health and fitness are in poor shape. It's imperative, and within your reach, to improve your health and fitness levels (not pop pills) to experience an effortless and regular period. The strategies below will help you improve body composition, lower body fat levels and improve insulin sensitivity and work at making the dream of a 'normal, pain-free period' a reality.

Note: Just like around menopause where your periods may naturally get irregular, scanty or heavy, it may also happen at menarche (first period). PCOS is something you may develop at any point of your 'reproductive age' (menarche to menopause). So make sure you learn to differentiate between the 'naturally' irregular period and the uncomfortable or the unnaturally irregular period. Also, natural or unnatural, these strategies will help.

To begin with, start lowering your body fat levels and make it easier for your ovaries to breathe, please. And no — stop hiding behind the excuse of PCOS/ PCOD. 'Lifestyle modification' is the buzzword here. Information is the key. Hopefully you have enough of the first buzzword to write a book now. So let's go to what can we do about it. As always, it's not about knowing, it's about doing.

Alright. Our strategies are based on improving insulin sensitivity (one of the reasons why you may be on 'diabetic medicine' if you have PCOS) and lowering body fat levels, the two main pillars of support for a healthy ovarian function. Easier said than done though, because it's going to take lot of work from your side.

Nutrition strategies

First things first, make time to eat, really. And if you have no time to eat, spare yourself the effort of reading further. Eating fresh food, wholesome food and eating in peace — you will need to do all these three, together, and at every meal, if you really care about your ovaries. If there is one thing that can really affect your whole life (health, body fat, looks, relationships — just about everything), it's the health of your ovaries. And the most important thing that plays a part in their health is nutrients and nutrient delivery — what you eat and whether it's reaching the ovaries. Simply put, do what you want, pop as many pills as you can lay your hands on, do laser wherever, but if you don't change your current eating (not eating) habits — babe, you're in a soup.

- So avoid soups. **Basically avoid anything that's overheated,** like an overcooked sabzi or dal that's boiled over and over, or plain reheated or microwaved food. Instead buy your veggies and fruits fresh and don't mash them into a juice or heat them into a soup. Preserve the nutrients by eating fresh.
- Don't go by the diet dictum of avoiding carbs. **With PCOS, you need carbs more than ever, and that too the unprocessed ones** like the humble wheat, rice, jowar, bajra, nachni or ragi, barley, etc. So please eat your roti, rotla, paratha, thalipeeth, thepla, dosa, etc. Whole grain carbs give us the much-needed fibre, which leads to a slow and steady rise of blood sugar (low GI) versus a sharp, fast rise in blood sugar (high GI or processed food). So give up on that 'low calorie sandwich' and eat your roti-sabzi or dal-chawal. Eat wholesome not half-hearted.

- The 'stuff' (hormones, enzymes, etc.) that affects (and gets affected by) our ovaries is all protein based, **so eating complete proteins is a must**. Which means that you can't be fussy and eat only salads: you will need to have dals, milk and milk-products, fish, eggs, paneer, cheese, etc. It's best to take it one step at a time. So to simplify things, begin by adding protein to the meal you have just before starting and ending the most active or stressful part of your day. So spice up your toast with an omelette or paratha with paneer for breakfast, and have a sprouts salad or cheese toast for an evening snack.

Seriously, improving protein intake is not half as complicated as it sounds. Simple acts like replacing colas with chaas or lassi will go a long way. Every amino acid (or lack of it) counts.

- **Stay away from everything that says 'fat-free' or 'low-fat' on the shelf.** Cut the fat from that upper abdomen and waist, not from your plate. Essential fatty acids like Omega-3 and Omega-6, which you can find in ghee, paneer and oils like groundnut, til, sesame, safflower, sunflower, rice bran, olive, coconut, etc., along with nuts, help decrease the glycemic index of the food. I know this is music to your ears — eating fat will slow down conversion of food to fat.

Snacks that are labelled 'low-fat' (FYI, they even sell low-fat butter) rob your body of essential fats, yes, but they also prevent absorption of fat-soluble vitamins like A, D and E. Now you need vitamin D for good bones and for that 'toned look'. And you need A and E for that fresh, supple skin, or at least to keep the acne from spreading.

And while we're talking about fat, have you heard of alpha lipoic acid (ALA)? Well, it's found in flaxseeds (alsi), walnuts and some green veggies. Now here's how it works — it mimics the action of insulin. So if insulin resistance is coming in the way of your fat loss, then all you need is to up your fat intake from sources that are rich in ALA. Btw, peas are rich in ALA too. With ALA in your diet, your body will actually find the nutritional support to pick up glucose (glucose uptake) and other nutrients from your blood stream.

- **Micro minerals like selenium, zinc and chromium improve our body's insulin sensitivity**. Simply put, it helps our pancreas secrete insulin in proportion to a rise in blood sugar. These are found in whole grains, so seriously, don't get swayed by the low-carb/low-fat diets, because you will only be compromising on essential nutrients that are actually helpful to ward off PCOS.

GTF or glucose tolerance factor (the name is self-explanatory; it's like when you hear 'Bond, James Bond', you know what to expect) is a vitamin-like substance that needs an adequate supply of chromium. Eat too many desserts, mithai, chocolate, sweets, and you compromise on your body's chromium stores. Now 'high insulin' or 'insulin resistance' depends on GTF and chromium is part of the GTF. So without GTF your insulin will not be able to pick up glucose from the cells. Insulin and GTF depend on each other and your metabolism depends on the efficiency of glucose uptake. Get it? No switching to nutrient-deprived cereals or 'enhanced' breads or late-night chocolate attacks. Just stick to the basics: **eat often, and eat often at home.**

- **Fresh curd, paneer, sprouts, idli, dosa (anything that's fermented) is priceless for ovaries because of the abundant supply of vitamin B12** (meats are a good source too). B12 plays a crucial role in iron absorption. Low haemoglobin levels are always a factor with irregular periods, lethargy, high body fat levels. Basically it's not uncommon to develop anaemia when you have irregular periods with heavy bleeding (common with PCOS).
- **Calcium is required 'more than normal'** in case you are experiencing PCOS. The cramps, headaches and general fatigue that you feel during periods or PMS will greatly reduce (and eventually stop) if you keep that supply of dietary calcium high. So move over tea at waking up, and late-night cappuccinos — pass the calcium tablet instead.

All-in-all, be a no-fuss girl and eat good food to help your body feel fresh, light and energetic. The hormones will respond by dancing freely and in perfect harmony.

Exercise strategies

1. The worst thing for irregular periods is irregular workouts. **Regular workouts are the key to regular periods.** A regular period means regular ovulation. Now purely from the point of getting pregnant, if you ovulate around twelve times a year, your chances of getting pregnant are much higher than if you ovulate (or get your periods) say four times a year. And purely from the point of getting thin and lean, regular period = hormonal

harmony = calm mind, good bone and muscle density = high BMR = low body fat levels = skinny jeans.

Regular ovulation which results in regular, effortless (without the help of a pill and without pain) period depends a lot on how oxygenated and nourished you keep your ovaries. Both oxygenation and nourishment depend on the blood circulation. Blood circulation depends on intelligent activity — read well-structured workouts.

2. Now it's important to not just structure your workout plan but to structure the 'workout', basically the time for it in your day. Too much? Okay, how about this: even seven days of workouts in a month done regularly over four to five months is much more helpful than twenty-five/thirty days of workouts in one month and then zero days in the next few months. Remember, *regularity* is the key here, and seven is a good number to start with. Then as you are able to stick with the seven days a month routine for three to four months, take it to fourteen days. And then again give yourself at least three months with the fourteen-day routine before multiplying the seven with three and taking it to twenty-one. **The point is not to be over-enthu, just be REGULAR.**

Oh, and it goes without saying, don't ever drop the number of workouts to lower than seven days a month. Read that again. I'm not saying seven *workouts* a month, I'm saying seven *days* a month. I know a lot of over-enthu people will not read properly and give me seven workouts a month by doing two-three workouts in one day. But by doing that, you are letting go of the all-important aspect of training your body to be regular. Got it?

3. **Weight-training workouts are a must** for two main reasons:

(a)They help strengthen all organs — heart, lungs, pancreas, ovaries and the entire involuntary system (that which is out of our control) ka team. Stronger organs means better efficiency. A stronger pancreas means better response of insulin (I keep coming back to this because PCOS has a strong link to insulin resistance or poor response from insulin) and stable blood sugar levels. Stable blood sugar means a much more intelligent use of fat as a fuel by your body. It also means a calmer, steadier, fresher mind. Wow, I have sold weight-training to myself once again and feel good already!

Stronger ovaries mean much more intelligent production of hormones like progesterone and estrogen — basically a much more harmonious situation for our hormones through the menstrual cycle. Hormones in harmony means less cramps during periods, no bloating or mood swings before periods, regular ovulation and an effortless period. Gosh! Why don't we all just quickly do a set of squats in gratitude to the many under-appreciated benefits of weight-training.

(b) After burn. Do you know what that means? See, we all know that when we go for a run, climb stairs, walk, etc. we burn calories, right? And we also burn calories at a rate higher than our basal or resting metabolic rate during exercise, right? Body fat is a major source of fuel for our resting metabolism, so in order to optimise fat burning, we ought to maximise our BMR or resting metabolic rate (basically optimise or max out fat burning during rest). Now after burn means that your body is burning fat at a rate higher than what it usually burns to keep your BMR going. The good news is that post weight-training, your body experiences an after burn for the next thirty-six to forty-eight hours (depending on the intensity of the workout, so do less time pass in the gym). Do the math: invest forty to sixty minutes in weight-training (burn calories during the workout, obviously) and then burn fat at a higher rate than normal for the next thirty-six to forty-eight hours. More after burn means lower body fat levels, lower body fat levels means less hormonal imbalances as high body fat disturbs the natural hormonal balance of the body, especially that of estrogens.

Okay, I know I said two main reasons, but I want to add one for the road. Weight-training leads to denser bones and stronger muscles — which means that sharp-toned body. Come on, move over bra fat (that which juts out from under the strap) and three-tyre stomach and jelly thighs — bring on that LBD.

Alright, so for best results, get regular with weight training and do it at least twice a week.

4. **Cardio is a great way to burn fat, especially if it's associated with learning new movements or a skill.** So how does a nice dance class or kick-boxing sound? Yes, yes, walking, jogging, swimming, cycling are good options too. But since you are going to be spending time burning calories, it just helps if you learn a new skill while you're at it (optimise time). Learning a new skill or art form means better nerve network per unit of muscle fibre (you know what I mean — it's the right hand can write but your left hand can barely hold the pen straight logic. Typically what gets used is what gets preserved and

improved upon by the body). Stronger nerve network leads to better strength in the body and helps improve blood circulation too.

5. Yogasanas are a brilliant way to bring about a balance in our entire system, and this balance easily reflects on our hormonal system too. Specifically, pelvic-opening asanas — those which help build strength and flexibility in our pelvic region — are great for our ovaries, and in fact our entire reproductive system, vagina included. Often, along with PCOS comes the bane of bloating, and what better to cure this than surya namaskars, which don't just help the lymphatic drainage, but stretch, flex and move the spine in its full range of movement to provide an excellent stimulation to all the organs (specifically the pancreas and the ovaries) to function to the best of their abilities. **Surya namaskars, along with pelvic-opening exercises, should form the basis of your asana practice**, but then again, be disciplined enough to learn all the basic postures and make your asana practice a holistic one by signing up with a sensible, patient and experienced teacher.

Weight-training, cardio with a skill and yogasanas are your options — you get to decide what form of exercise you would like to practise more often. If you are going by the minimum seven-day rule, you can spend two days on each of the forms and repeat your favourite on the extra day.

Sleep strategies

As is the case with workouts, with sleep too regularity is the key. **Sleep at the same time every day and wake up at the same time every day if you are really keen on**

staying hormonally vibrant. Irregular bed times and, worse, mails, phone calls, TV before going to sleep, can wreak havoc on your hormones if they are already feeling a bit 'off'. And remember what I told you about IGF-1 and sleep in the Hypothyroid chapter? Well, that applies for PCOS too (ya, ya, all hormones in our body are interlinked — if one of them is disturbed or out of balance, then the entire hormonal system is disturbed). IGF-1 and insulin sensitivity is strongly connected or interlinked, so if there's one thing you can't compromise on, it's sleep. Also remember, an effortless period (regular) is not an isolated incident, it is simply a manifestation of regularity in your lifestyle. A restorative and peaceful sleep is also crucial for the absorption of minerals like calcium and iron, both of which run low in case of hormonal imbalances or PCOS. A regular bedtime hour prepares the body to fall into deep sleep and brings about a calming effect on the body and mind, which leads to a sense of harmony for the hormones. An irregular bedtime has the exact opposite effect on hormones — they feel agitated. Late nights also mean a bloated body and sugar cravings the next morning, and you totally don't want that. And just like workouts, it's not like having those eight hours of sleep once in a while, but the regularity of that eight-hour sleep that matters.

Relationship strategies

Typically, an imbalance in hormones wreak havoc in interpersonal relationships (unstable blood sugars leading to irritability, mood swings and low self-esteem).

If you find yourself in a relationship where you are taking on more than your share of responsibilities, trust me, your hormones will protest. PCOS (and high prolactin or endometriosis) is simply one of the ways that your hormones are asking you to balance out or share your burden. PCOS/PCOD is an urban phenomenon and common amongst girls and women who have that spark of brilliance and want more out of life. Very often women feel guilty simply because they are achievers (or competitive) at work or college, and they start by compensating for this by doing more than they should, or even more frequently compromising on more than they should be with their husbands/boyfriends. Reasserting your right to lead a complete life or to be an achiever is a big step forward. It's okay to be smarter than the lot, it's not a crime, chill.

The tantric philosophy talks about balance between Shiva and Shakti or male and female energies or that of yin and yang that flow through our body. The analytical abilities, extrovert nature or action-oriented nature is due to the 'masculine energy'. If a woman is in awe of her abilities to think, rationalise and act, then she super compensates by overworking the 'feminine energy'. Some women (mostly older) do it by overtly complying to the 'ideal woman' image of doing everything at home and spoon-feeding husband, children, in-laws, to the extent where they completely run out of energy (almost depression). Others (mostly younger) do it by trying to suppress their femininity (beauty is a virtue of 'female energy') and by 'being the man', or they try and act harsh and cold (manly) even though they may feel warm and friendly from inside. Under-dressing or dressing in a way that almost reduces their beauty is another form of expressing the need to block out the feminine aspect of energy.

Now the problem is that if you under-work or overwork the feminine aspect, you are bound to land in trouble because it creates an imbalance in the masculine and feminine aspects of energy. So learn to express yourself freely and fearlessly. The more you allow uninterrupted or undisturbed flow of energies, the more likely are you to find a balance not just in your energies, but also in your hormones and life itself.

You've heard of the seven chakras? Swadhisthana is the chakra in your genital area and the reproductive system is said to vibrate here. It is supposed to be the chakra for sex, power, money and to all the worldly pleasures of life. It's also linked strongly to creativity (and therefore pregnancy or ability to reproduce). Being at peace with one's sexuality and understanding yourself sexually is one of the ways of liberating yourself from the whole hormonal imbalance drama. Most city folk are tight at their hip or pelvic joints because they either don't fully understand or have enough of sex, power and money. Once you learn to channelise the pleasure part (sex, power, money) of the chakra, the creativity aspect of the chakra begins to bloom. For creativity to flow uninterruptedly you must find that sense of calm and peace in your mind, body and hormones. Creativity also flows when you spend time with yourself learning or understanding your worldly needs and your spiritual needs. Again, to lead a complete life, you will need to seek and gain that all-important balance between your worldly and spiritual pursuits.

Real life diet analysis

Seema Mishra is a forty-year-old housewife who has just given up her job at a bank after eighteen years.

She suffers from a mild form of Polycystic Ovarian Syndrome, resulting in insulin resistance. She has been taking four tablets of Glucophage (500mg) a day (one each after breakfast, lunch, tea and dinner). Sometimes she takes two after dinner. She also takes four tablets of Aldactone (25mg; two at breakfast and two at dinner).

With the diet she was on, she was restricted from having carbs and advised not to eat roti, rice, potatoes, sweets. She does not like this high-protein, low-carb diet (she does not enjoy eating chicken but did so because she felt she 'needed' to). She finds it very difficult to adhere to this on a day-to-day basis and feels terribly guilty every time she slips up or 'eats like us Indians'.

Three-day diet recall

Time	Food/ Drink	Activity Recall	Workout
Day 1			
4.45 a.m.	2 glasses of water (one after another)	Woke up, went to the washroom, freshened up	
5.15 – 6.00 a.m.			Did pranayam, surya namaskars (10), kapalbhati (600 times), brahmri, Bhastrika

6.30 a.m.	1 bowl of sweet melon		
7.00 a.m.		Dropped my daughter to the bus stop and went to the gym	
7.15 – 8.00 a.m.			Worked out in the gym
8.30 a.m.		Showered and dressed	
8.45 a.m.	1 boiled egg, 1 multigrain high fibre cracker (low carbs), half cup coffee (made with ¼ cup lacto-free milk and ½ cup water) with sweetener		
9.15 – 11.30 a.m.		Attended a job interview. Drove to venue and back	
11.45 a.m.	1 small bowl of salad with capsicum, cucumber, carrot, moong sprouts and lettuce leaves with 1 tbsp light Italian dressing		
11.45 – 12.30 p.m.		Chatted on the phone with ex-colleagues	
12.30 – 1.00 p.m.	One glass water		Ran on treadmill for half an hour at 5.5 miles an hour
1.30 p.m.		Showered again	
1.45 p.m.	1½ cups rice with sukhi prawns, potatoes and cabbage	Feeling guilty as I want to avoid carbs, but when it's prawns it's gotta be rice! God help me!!	
2.00 – 4.00 p.m.		Watched TV	

4.00 p.m.	Half cup tea made with lacto-free milk with 2 tablets sweetener		
4.00 – 6.00 p.m.		Taught my son	
6.00 p.m.	Half Atkins chocolate protein bar (consisting of 8.5 gms of protein)		
6.15 – 8.30 p.m.		Took my daughter for the Speedo swimming class. Drove approx 12 km one way, waited there and drove back	
8.30 p.m.	Had 1 glass of water followed with 1 flour tortilla (carbs 13 gms) + 1 leg of chicken curry, had 1 tsp of sweet boondi (prasad from temple)		
9.30 p.m.		Went to sleep	
Day 2			
4.45 a.m.	2 glasses of water (one after another)	Woke up	
5.15 – 6.00 a.m.			Did pranayam, surya namaskar (80; 20 slow, 60 fast) and asanas for legs
6.30 a.m.	Bowl of sweet melon		
7.00 a.m.		Dropped my daughter to the bus stop	
7.30 – 8.30 a.m.			Bharat Thakur yoga class
9.00 a.m.		Showered and dressed	

9.30 a.m.	1 whole egg omelette, 1 glass lassi made with full cream, yogurt and sweetener	Picked up my daughter from school and brought her home	
10.00 – 10.30 a.m.		Went to Evision counter (300m walking)	
11.00 – 11.30 a.m.		Went to dentist (drove 2 km and back)	
11.30 a.m.	1 glass of water, 1 small bowl of salad with capsicum, cucumber, moong sprouts and lettuce leaves with 1 tbsp Thousand Island dressing		
11.45 a.m. – 1.30 p.m.		Went to hair salon for hair colour touch up, (drove approx 1 km and back)	
1.45 p.m.	1 glass of water, 1 flour tortilla with a small bowl of lauki kofta curry, 1 small bowl of boondi raita		
2.00 – 4.00 p.m.		Watched TV	
4.00 p.m.	Half cup tea made with lacto-free milk with 2 tablets sweetener		
4.00 – 6.00 p.m.		Taught my son	
6.00 p.m.	Atkins chocolate protein bar (consisting of 17 gms of protein)		
6.15 p.m.		Climbed 3 floors to visit friend in building	

8.30 p.m.	Had 1 glass of water followed with a small bowl of palak paneer	Took daughter for a class	
9.30 p.m.		Went to sleep	
Day 3 (Holiday)			
7. 15 a.m.	2 glasses of water (one after another)	Woke up	
7.45 a.m.	Half cup tea made with lacto-free milk with 2 tablets sweetener		
8.30 a.m.			Went to gym
9.30 a.m.		Showered and dressed	
10.00 a.m.		Took my son for French tuition. Walked 200m and back	
10.30 a.m.	1 whole egg scrambled, 4 mushrooms (sauteed in butter, garlic, salt and pepper), 1 chicken sausage boiled and fried), half cup coffee made with lacto-free milk with 2 tablets sweetener		
11.00 a.m.		Went to pick up my son from tuition. Walked 200m and back	
11.30 a.m. – 12.15 p.m.		Took my son for a dance class	
1.00 p.m.	1 glass water, a few pieces of paneer tikka and chicken tikka, salad with capsicum, cucumber, carrot		

2.00 – 5.00 p.m.		Watched movie in a movie hall	
3.00 p.m.	Atkins chocolate protein bar (consisting of 17 gms of protein)		
5.30 p.m.	Had tea and nuts		
6.00 – 7.30 p.m.		Cooked 3 dishes	
8.30 p.m.	Had a few pieces of paneer tikka and chicken tikka kabab, along with 1 Diet Coke		
9.00 – 10.00 p.m.		Watched TV	
10.00 p.m.		Went to sleep	

Evaluation of the recall

Seema is making an effort to eat what she thinks is healthy because she has been advised to do so.

Looking at her recall, you can see that she is doing a lot through the day: exercising, taking care of the kids, driving, cooking. At the same time she is making an effort to stick to her low-carb, high-protein diet. In the process, she is starving herself to an extent.

If, instead of eliminating carbs, she eats complete meals of carbs, protein, fats with the right balance of vitamins, minerals and water, she will feel more satisfied with her meals and her insulin response will improve (poor insulin response is a precursor to PCOS).

When carbohydrates are not adequately present in the diet, then the body starts using protein (and later also fat) as a source of energy and therefore proteins will not be present in sufficient amount to perform their important functions, such as rebuilding damaged tissues, building muscles, transporting nutrients, producing hormones, enzymes, etc.

So being on a low-carb diet is in no way improving her insulin response. In fact, because she eats like this, the cells are always starved as they do not receive the nutrients they need. In the absence of adequate carbs, insulin is unable to do this important job of carrying the nutrients to the cells. Fats and proteins, when combined with the right carbohydrates, slow down the release of blood sugar and improve insulin response.

The good part about this recall is that Seema is very regular with her exercise. This is definitely helping her improve her fitness levels, but she needs to eat more wholesome food through the day so that she gets the maximum benefit from her food and exercise.

Modifications

If Seema is more careful about her food and makes an attempt to eat right (not what she thinks is right, but what is actually right for her body) her insulin response will improve (and therefore the PCOS). She will also lose fat and not go through mood swings (a by-product of PCOS and low-carb diets) like she does right now.

The diet recommended for Seema was as below:

Meal 1 (6.00 a.m., after pranayam): Muesli + milk

Meal 2 (8.00 a.m.): 2 egg whites + whole wheat toast

Meal 3 (10.00 a.m.): Laban/chaas

Meal 4 (12.00 p.m.): Poha/upma/idli-sambhar + chutney (she had been depriving herself of 'good food' and didn't have the time in the morning to cook these as traditional breakfast items. She loved it that her 'off time' from jobs presented her with the opportunity to cook and eat — GUILT-free — and that too when no one was at home, so peacefully!)

Meal 5 (2.00 p.m.): Handful of peanuts

Meal 6 (4.00 p.m.): Cheese

Meal 7 (6.00 p.m.): Roti + green sabzi + dal or kadhi

Meal 8 (8.00 p.m.): Glass of warm milk

Seema adapted to this eating pattern and followed the diet to a T.

Her diet was changed regularly to bring in different food options so as to expose her body to different nutrients. She was also asked to take vitamin B-complex, vitamin C, calcium, flaxseeds, zinc and magnesium supplements, as each of these minerals and vitamins plays a role in regulating hormonal action.

She was very regular and disciplined with her exercise as well. (In fact, she was over-exercising in her bid to lose weight. Overexercising reduces fat burning and leads to fatigue and further hormonal imbalances.) PCOS has a strong link to stress. So though she had quit her job for the time being, she was 'utilising' her time by over-exercising. Physical stress is as harmful as mental stress. She was advised to work out only once a day, instead of twice.

Six weeks after these changes were made, she completely stopped taking the Aldactone. After eight weeks, she was able to reduce the Glucophage to three tablets a day.

By this time she was already looking more toned, feeling much better in terms of her energy levels, her skin was glowing and her exercise performance had improved.

After another eight weeks, she completely stopped the Glucophage.

After all these changes, Seema feels and looks younger than ever before, her skin is glowing more than it has ever before, and she does not feel fatigued at the end of the day. In fact, she feels much more energetic and her exercise performance has also gotten better.

Her periods are regular, pain-free and actually enjoyable — a sign that insulin resistance and PCOS is now history!

Some dope on medicine

Every drug that has an effect has a side effect. That's a rule nobody can deny. If the pill that you are taking for PCOS/ hypothyroid/ diabetes/high blood pressure is 'good' for you, then its goodness is also going to do something not-so-good, in fact bad, for you. Only when the 'bad' or side effect is clearly visible do we sit up and take notice: like a rash post an antibiotic will make you think twice about the antibiotic. You will avoid it as much as you can and take it only when you really need to (when you think the benefits of the antibiotic is worth the inconvenience of the rash).

That's the logic we need to apply before taking drugs to 'treat' our 'condition', even if the side effects are not as visible as the rash on the skin. Most of the drugs disturb your intestines, your inner or intimate skin. The medicines that you may be taking for PCOS lead to mal-absorption of the (any guesses?) all-important vitamin B12. Now B12 is involved in some of the really crucial metabolic processes: it is involved in keeping your heart healthy, making your haemoglobin, utilising your carbs right (keeping your energy levels high), helping your neurotransmitters along with B6 and other B vitamins, etc. Very specifically for PCOS, it is involved in reducing elevated levels of homcysteine (an amino acid found in the blood).

High levels of homocysteine (normal levels are not a problem) are associated with pregnancy complications, chronic fatigue syndrome, high blood pressure, heart diseases, etc. Basically it's an indicator of malfunctioning metabolic processes. If you have PCOS, your homocysteine levels are likely to be high (your requirement of vitamin B including B12 is higher than normal), and with the drugs you take for PCOS, it's at a risk of elevating further (mal-absorption of B12) — keeping you in that loop of 'low energy, mood swings, risk of developing high blood pressure, bloating, pregnancy complications' forever.

The thing to do is to understand all the side effects of the effective drug that you are taking as 'treatment'. Is the benefit worth the risk? Popping a pill without doing your risk-benefit analysis is, well, risky.

Know your medicine. I find a lot of my clients not even knowing what they are taking. Like a fourteen-year-old who was on contraceptives but didn't know that she was on one. She thought of it as just 'medicine'. Of course she felt worse day by day, becoming a 'difficult child' for her mother to handle and having some serious mood swings even in school (mood swings are a well-documented side effect of oral contraceptives). Even her mom didn't associate her 'rude' behaviour with the 'medicine'; basically the whole family was in the dark about their little girl being on contraceptives and thought of her change in behaviour as tantrums of today's generation, exam stress, etc. Then there was this forty-six-year-old client who was put on medication for 'low energy' and it turned out to be anti-depressants. She was clueless that she was on anti-depressants, she just thought it was medicine to feel energetic and wondered why she felt sleepy all day in office. Just because something is given to you as 'medicine' or as something 'good for you' doesn't take away your right to know what that medicine is all about. Knowing and understanding what you are taking and exposing your body to it is completely your responsibility. If the medicine doesn't suit you and you tell your doctor about it, she won't beat you up or think you are rude/ disrespectful, etc. She may offer you an alternative or change the line of treatment, but give her the chance to know that it's not working for you.

For how long should you take it. The other thing is going on with a medicine forever. A sixty-six-year-old client of mine was on a strong anti-anxiety medicine. Have you been prescribed this, I asked. Well my doctor had asked me to take it for the first flight I took because I was very nervous. When did you take the flight? When I was forty years old. Wow! Does your doctor know that you are still taking it? Ladies, the doctor was as shocked as I was — this lady was supposed to take the drug for just one week.

4

The Four Strategies For Well-Being

I

Nutrition Strategies

Food sustains the life of living beings. All living beings in the universe require food. Complexion, clarity, good voice, longevity, genius, happiness, satisfaction, nourishment, strength and intellect are all conditioned by food.

–*Charak Samhita*

I was digging into my bowl of fresh fruit, debating whether the 1600m height at Katrain (near Manali) really qualified as altitude. I had given up after just two kilometres of running along the Beas, had tweeted, 'Running along the Beas — the altitude just killed me and the sheer beauty is putting life back into me', and was mindlessly chewing (yes, guilty) my fruits. An unusually crisp, juicy and refreshingly (almost heady) sweet taste brought my attention back to the act of 'eating'. Hmm ... what fruit is this, I wondered. I have always eaten a wide variety of fruits, and I take pride in my ability to recognise the mildest of flavours, aromas, taste, etc. I mean, I have a sharp tongue, literally and figuratively.

So I called on my memory to match this taste, what this fruit was that I was chewing on. It was familiar and distinct and yet not traceable. My inability to 'know' what I was eating teased my mind. I took another bite, chewed it slowly, closed my eyes, opened my mouth wide on finishing and inhaled through my mouth and now used sight, sound, smell, touch, taste, everything I could, to figure out this fruit. Okay, surely it's something local that I've never eaten in my life, I told myself, and marched towards the kitchen.

'Yeh kaunsa fruit hai?' I asked with great curiosity, holding the mysterious piece of fruit in my hand.

'Yeh?' said Bobby (the guy on morning duty) dismissively. 'Pear.'

What? I have eaten pears all my life. I took a bite again — god! It was indeed pear. And it didn't even taste like one. It tasted magical, almost divine, enticing me to use more than one of my sense organs to unravel it, and teasing my curiosity without once revealing its true identity.

So why hadn't I recognised it? Simple. I had NEVER eaten it at its place of origin! So my memory or recognition of a 'pear' was a compromised experience. And trust me, I have eaten good pears, bought them from the best of markets, bought them fresh, eaten them without cutting them into pieces, relished every bite and generally done all I can to get the most out of my fruit. I had overlooked the most crucial aspect though — the pears I'd eaten had always been off the tree for days, maybe weeks before they reached the Vashi market from where they enter other smaller markets of Mumbai. During this long and often tiring, uncomfortable journey, the pear had lost its crisp, fresh taste, the colour of its skin had faded, even become black at a few places because of the friction with other pears. With many of its vitamins, bioflavonoids and micro minerals lost, it didn't taste anything like it really should.

Now imagine having a pear which had literally grown ten meters away from where I'd ended my jog, and add to that the fact that it was living on a tree minutes before its consumption. So as my tongue and all other sense organs revelled in its freshness and magical taste, it blessed my digestive system with its mineral, fibre, vitamin and enzyme-rich presence, raising my blood sugar just enough to motivate my insulin to carry all the goodness to my starving cells. Ah! The feeling, the blessing of eating fresh!

And now to weight loss. Why talk of eating fresh? Simply because the better your nourishment status, the better your digestion; the better the digestion, better the assimilation; better the assimilation (and excretion), better the health; better the health, better the fatburning mechanism of the body; better the fat-burning mechanism (metabolism) of the body, slimmer the waist.

This really is the mainstay of our Nutrition strategies:

1. Eat local, think global
2. Portion size
3. Food planning
4. Beyond calories

1. Eat local, think global

To think big, to think global, to think beyond your limitations, the body must be well-nourished, the mind must be calm. Well that's possible only if the food is richer calorie to calorie, or in non-layman terms, high nutrient to calorie ratio. So theoretically, if you get a hundred calories per pear in Mumbai and a hundred calories per pear in its place of origin, which pear will give you a slimmer waist? I'll give you a hundred rupees if you get the answer wrong.

Food miles

Here's a simplified correlation for you: **the longer your food travelled before landing on your plate (food miles), the longer your navel will travel away from your spine.** Bole ga toh — big fat stomach, three-tyre system.

Eating local and what is in season (lower food miles) helps bring the navel closer to the spine and lifts your butt up as well. Also, what grows around the place you stay is equipped to safeguard you against all the environmental challenges that you face. For example, food that grows around the coastal area in an iodine-rich soil condition (kelp, the sea vegetable, is a great source) helps to keep your thyroid healthy. And please can we treat our bananas, chickoo, seetaphal, jackfruit, grapefruit, oranges, etc. a little better now? Chickoo from Gholvad, santra from Nagpur, walnut from Kashmir, apple from Kinnaur, jackfruit from Konkan, guava from Pune, grapes from Nasik, bananas from Kerala — humble origins, exotic results. Or are we going to wait for the West to go gaga over them before learning to accept that these are good for us (we have done it with yoga, we almost did it with turmeric, basmati and cow urine).

So now what? Don't eat those exotic cranberries, prunes from California, olive oil from Italy, the 'English vegetable' from London, the apple from New Zealand and all the 'rich' stuff? Hello! Have it. I am not on a swadeshi morcha. All that I'm saying is that what grows in California will taste and assimilate better in California.

So eat all the exotic stuff, but not at the cost of not eating what grows locally. So another equation: five days of the week eat local or food that has travelled fewer miles, and on two days you can indulge your 'exotic tooth'.

GI

Heard of 'Geographical Identification'? GI is similar to a trademark or an intellectual property. So now we have proper recognition of Darjeeling tea, Banarasi silk, Tirupati laddoo, Goan feni and soon perhaps Hyderabadi haleem. It's a validation of the fact that tea that grows in Darjeeling is unique in its properties, taste, texture, flavour, aroma (read nutrients, discovered and yet to be discovered), and that this uniqueness brings with it advantages to the gastrointestinal tract or our digestive system that are unique and desirable. Needless to add, removing the foods from their native location does reduce their properties, even if it means their consumption just outside their geographic territory. Now just because Kerala banana or your gaon ka local fruit hasn't earned a GI yet doesn't make it less important or exotic. So please learn to value its uniqueness.

2. Portion size

Eating local and eating in season appeals to our common sense, but how much should we eat? Can I eat all I want just because it's local and rich in nutrients; won't I put on weight if I overdo it? Arrey, I know what you want to hear (read) — NO. You won't gain weight. **Mitahar means**

eating with all your senses, eating healthy (local) and eating in peace, which will ensure that you eat the right quantity. The quantity of food you consume should be dictated only by your stomach and not by a dietician (or trainer/doctor/mother/any health professional), the latest fad or much less the fear of getting fat. Our shastras say that the wise man knows when to stop eating and the fool always overeats. Now how do you know if you have overeaten? You know it when you experience discomfort or pain later. This discomfort becomes a part of our life, but instead of learning from our pain (yes, pain is our friend), we strangle it with meds, antacids, 'ayurvedic' pills and all the duniya bhar ka kachara. But do we learn to eat till a point where we feel calm, easy, light? No, we learn to 'deal' with the pain of routinely overeating.

There is a saying: if you don't learn from history, history will repeat itself. So if you don't learn from overeating, overeating will repeat itself. Eventually you will lose confidence in yourself, in your ability to decide what to eat, how much to eat, when to eat (and stop), etc. Enter the weight loss industry — toning table, belts, pills, surgeries, low cal food, pre-packaged meals, gym, trainers, dieticians (ya, it's a multimillion-dollar industry out there). The industry thrives on your feelings of inadequacy: you're not thin enough, fit enough, beautiful enough, flat enough on your stomach, round enough on your breasts, etc. Okay, forget it, I am digressing again, but why did I even digress? Because it's relevant to the 'portion' or size of your meal.

See it's basically like this: overeat and it leads to discomfort and pain, with that comes fear. So you stay away from food or starve after an episode of overeating. Now here's the flipside: the other side of the fear coin is greed, so at the next meal you overeat again. Now you're running up and down the bridge which leads from fear to greed; you overeat, you starve, you feast, you fast, you dabbao, you go into a 'can't even look at food' mode again. I so wish this was a vicious cycle, but it's really a downward spiral — at the very bottom of which is fad diets which enforce starvation-like conditions (I mean, please, if you are so averse to eating, just exchange places with one person from the forty per cent of our population that don't get even two meals a day; then at least you can justify the torture you put your body though every time you 'decide' to 'lose weight'), or putting your body through pills, needles, surgeries and a host of other 'quick and guaranteed' methods. And yes, depression, loss of confidence and the host of obesity-related diseases just come with it; package deal, girls.

When you run from one end of the bridge to the other, fear to greed, greed to fear, you feel out of breath, out of shape, and out of your mind! Not surprising, na? So then what? S - I - M - P - L - E, that's what my three-year-old nephew Sunay says every time he finds the right piece in a jigsaw puzzle. The missing piece here is making time to eat in peace. When you eat in peace (not in pieces, with your attention also on work, remote control, phone, god knows millions of other things), then you will hear your stomach talk to you. It speaks in a language each one of us, rich or poor, educated or illiterate, fat or thin, married or unmarried, happy or sad, can understand.

Things you can do to ensure you eat the right quantity:

a) The rule of UNO

Have you played Uno? If you have, you know the rules — when you have just one card left, you're supposed to say 'Uno', or else you've missed your chance and are forced to pick another card from the pack, and that one card can turn your winning streak into a losing one.

Guess you're getting where this is leading. When there is still a bit of space left in your stomach, it says 'Uno'. If you are alert enough to hear that, you put a full stop to your game of eating. If you didn't hear your stomach say Uno, or you heard and chose to ignore it (or you were just 'busy'), then you pick up another morsel and lose at the game of eating 'right', looking thin, staying fit, healthy, happy, calm. Congratulations. And no amount of 'working out tomorrow' or 'slogging at the treadmill tomorrow' is going to change that — you are doomed to stay trapped on the bridge that leads you from greed to fear. To escape the bridge, simply listen, *listen* to your stomach.

Now the stomach will say 'Uno' at different times during different phases of our growth and menstrual cycle. When it says 'Uno' is also dependent on your stress- levels (mental and physical), the time of day, season, geographical location, company during meals and a host of other factors. Women should never, ever (saying this at the cost of knowing never say never) 'standardise' their meal size. **We are hormonally vibrant, and it's perfectly NORMAL to feel like eating more on some days and less on other days**. The key is to stop at the right time. Oh, btw, even our genes can determine the stomach's capacity.

Overeating disturbs not just our feeling of well-being, sense of calm and pride (yes, people; there is a sense of dignified pride in stopping at 'Uno', trust me), but also the hormonal balance, specifically that of serotonin (now emerging as a strong link to appetite control) and insulin (obvious, isn't it?), our satiety centre and of course our

blood circulation (that's why we feel so numbed, all we want to do is sleep). And believe me, as counterintuitive as it may sound, it's really difficult to overeat. Yes, you heard (read) right, it's DIFFICULT to overeat and EFFORTLESS to eat right. The only reason that we manage to overeat all the time is because, as 'modern' women, we are fast losing our ability to rely on our intuition, much less nurture or value it.

b) Gut feeling

What is listening to your stomach? A gut instinct? Intuition?

The reason why women have been more spiritual than men since time immemorial is because they are gifted or blessed with the power of intuition. Our ancient scriptures tell all of us to be fearless. You get that — be fearless, listen to your own voice and learn to stop eating at the right point. What do we do instead? Listen to our friends, mother-in-law, well-meaning relatives who goad us into eating more ('one day you can eat more/ek din khane se kuch nahi hota/a little mithai is not going to make you into a hippo/oh come on, be a sport have another one/don't be so stuck-up, etc.'). I have been working since 1999, and I have NEVER met a person who didn't know that she was overeating. I have often been privy to conversations that sound like: 'I knew if I ate another roti then I would be stuffed, but I don't know why, I just did it because I wanted my MiL/people to stop talking about my "diet", and after that I don't know what happened I just had a jalebi and then a malai sandwich — full throttle. Now I feel like shit.'

The next time somebody goads you to eat a little more, ask them if they will share your burden of overeating, of hormones going for a toss, of the brain being drained of blood, of insulin being overworked, of fat cells getting bigger, of feeling fatigued, of your heart rate and breathing rate going up, of organs feeling squeezed under fat cells. If they answer in the positive, then maybe, just maybe you can do it. Remember the story in the *Ramayan*, when Valya is asked by Narada if his parents, wife and children will share his karma of being a robber and killing people? His family refused, and Valya became Valmiki. Apna karma share karne ke liye koi nahi aata hai, boss. So overeat at your own risk and discretion.

c) Eating small

Probably the most misunderstood concept by all those who want to eat right. Once you start practising the four principles of eating right (see Introduction), your meal size may naturally drop or become smaller as a consequence of eating every two hours. But that's not the agenda, really. The agenda is to stay tuned to your stomach and fearlessly eat what it requires. So on a day when you feel like one roti, eat one; when you feel like five, eat five; when you feel like half, eat half. Just make sure you are not crossing the overeating threshold or disrespecting the

'Uno' signal. **Eating right is not about having a 'small portion', but the *right* portion.** And only you can decide what the right portion is for yourself. This is exactly what I tell my clients — as a nutritionist I will help you with what nutrients you need and at what time (based on diet and activity recall). As a person who wants to stay lean and fit for life, it's *your* job to consume the right quantity — not more, not less. Aim to feel light and energetic post a meal, not stuffed and dull.

The one thing that hurts me a lot is to see how my clients who have been to all the dieticians and diets and weight loss programmes in the world still struggle with their weight (because of the yo-yo effect) and lose faith in their ability to know the right amount to eat. Some of them have even asked me to return their money for refusing to 'fix' their portions. 'I just want to eat exactly what you tell me,' said an exasperated client. 'I want to give getting thin a chance.' Well, you stand a chance to get and stay thin only if you listen to your stomach and not me. If I fix your quantity because you don't want to use your brains (ya, she said; if she had to use her brains in deciding how much to eat, then why pay a dietician), then it's going to be a disaster for both of us. For her, because with me restricting her portion, she can eat 'small' for a while, but what after that? She goes back to eating big because she didn't learn to listen to her stomach. Then she may need another diet/dietician/weight loss programme, so it's a never-ending story. For me it's a failure because she would be a client who gained weight post her diet with me. I rate my programme's success based on what clients learn and how well they learn to listen to their stomach, and not on how much weight they lose.

Appetite

Hunger is a sign of youth and health, loss of appetite, a sign of disease or loss of youth. So nurture your appetite (possible only by eating right) and eating well. Often when I am in the Himalaya for a yoga course, I am amazed at how our genes too play such a large role in our appetites. Even though we all do the same activity, have the same sleep and wake-up times, I find that my Caucasian friends typically eat much more than I do and are just as strong, lean and fit (if not more) as my Asian friends who eat less than them and a little more than me. So it's really not the quantity, it's about whether you are eating 'right' for your requirements and your ability to digest, assimilate, excrete.

It's time to throw away the math we have been fed: calories in = calories out (no weight gain)/calories in > calories out (weight gain)/calories in < calories out (weight loss). Weight gain, loss, maintenance, whatever you are trying to achieve goes beyond maths. It involves the history of your meal pattern and workout status, geography of the place you are currently in — climate, humidity, etc., the molecular chemistry of how the food you are eating is responding with your enzymes, hormones, etc., and above all, the state of your mind. It may sound like the 'it's complicated' Facebook status, but it's not, it's actually rather simple. The point is to keep your focus on the simplest and most obvious part of the equation: are you hungry? Do you feel like you have a good appetite? If the answer is yes, girl you're on track. You're getting fitter, stronger, leaner (ya, losing weight too), and looking like a million bucks! Just keep feeding that fire in your stomach.

3. Food planning

Failing to plan is planning to fail — whoever said this knew how to get the maximum effect from minimum words. Planning to eat right is a bit like that — learning to get the max out of food with minimum effort and tenshun (that's Marathi for tension). So here's the one strategy that you should learn: always plan today what you will be eating tomorrow.

We are becoming experts at planning backwards: self-help books goad us to plan our funeral first and life later. Now if we were to think of our body as the finished product, then the building material or raw product is what we put in it. I'm sure you all know that the quality of the finished product depends on the quality of the raw material, right? So eating local will help keep the raw material fresh, and eating the right quantity helps us to optimally absorb the freshness and goodness of local produce. Now what about the quality of local produce? That's the point I would like to discuss while talking about food planning. All of us want to look fresh and glowing, and be energetic, thin and toned. For that to be possible, we need to go deeper than the maths of calories and look at how our food is grown and nurtured, along the railway tracks or under the watchful eye of a knowledgeable farmer in an unpolluted village on a fertile land that he tills with care, love and compassion?

Food quality

In India, we've traditionally had the practice of storing a year's stock of grains, pulses, spices and condiments that we regularly use. This activity is usually undertaken during summer when the food is first 'sun dried' to fortify the food and as step one of getting it ready to be stored. It's cleaned meticulously, and the storage area is purified and disinfected using indigenous methods and natural products.

No, I am not telling you this to make you feel guilty or to tell you to do behenji giri; all I'm saying is that women spent a lot of time with their food before it came on their plate. And during this time a lot of quality control measures were undertaken. Typically, they also had a fair idea about which field or place their food came from. This means they were quite in the loop about the soil conditions, farm yield that year, the unseasonal showers, the mode of transport used for their food and probably even names, faces and life histories of the people who actually grew their food. You can compare this to wanting to be in the know of the school (schooling and teachers) that your kids study in. We spend time and diligently mark PTA meetings on our calendars, meet other mothers for coffee/lunch or volunteer to do work in school, all to ensure that the quality of education is up to our expectation and because we believe that being involved in the process helps both us and our children grow. We don't think of this as too difficult/downmarket/cheap/behenji types or only for the poor; rather we practically glorify it and take pride in our involvement. Same reasons to get involved with your food and the whole process.

The point is, if food is just landing on your plate and at the most you know which supermarket you picked it up from, then it's like your kid dropping in at home to say she is going from Class 5 to Class 6. Your involvement is close to zero and therefore your control or ability to tell if any learning actually happened is ZERO. Similarly, your ability to tell if your food is nourishing is close to zero. Little wonder then that you eat and feel tired or feel the need to drink tea/coffee/have a cigarette/small piece of chocolate post your meal. Food fails to nourish or energise you; it's almost depleting your energy levels, in some cases actually making you feel dull and drowsy.

Farmers' markets

This is a concept that's big in the world's biggest and bestest city — New York. It's not a concept, it's actually a huge movement, much like the traditional bazaars that India has always had. The Wednesday bazaar or the Sunday bazaar. In fact, small town and rural India is still blessed with bazaars. I just hope we don't lose this tradition to 'development and progress' and then have NY or the West at large reintroduce it to us in a grand, cool way.

So a weekly bazaar is a fixed day when farmers in the locality come to a fixed place and sell their produce. You get the best of sabzi, fruits, grains, dry fruits and at reasonable prices. Good for all. Also it's a great place to bond, socialise and gossip. It's almost a movement in New York: these weekly markets are held in Madison Park, Union Park, Central Park, and loads of other places in the city. So you will have farmers from upstate and NJ selling their stuff and city folk relishing the experience. They even have the best of chefs in the city volunteer to help the 'green movement' by sharing and teaching the crowds how to cook using fresh ingredients to retain flavours and aromas of the foods, and turning them into yummy, healthy dishes. They hand out flyers teaching buyers how to store the food.

In India we know these things, they are a part of our DNA — and if we don't use them we will lose them.

God! Sorry for making your food sound like a nightmare, **but here's what you can do to ensure that**

food nourishes and doesn't deplete. Moving back to your village is not what I am suggesting (though that's not a bad idea either).

- Involve your family and make 'know your kitchen' a non-negotiable family activity.
- Typically, just outside of your city toll naka, you will find farms from where you can buy stuff like dals, wheat, rice, other coarse grains you like — ragi, jowar, bajra. Middleman out, both you and the farmer will benefit. You know a face you can relate to and can ensure that transport is cleaner and faster too.
- This immediately adds value, goodness and freshness to your food. It's time-consuming, and takes effort and planning, but it is truly a rewarding experience, worth every bit of the trouble.
- If this is not possible, pool your resources with a group of like-minded friends and buy some land and learn to grow your food. Don't worry, human resources are plenty in our country and you will learn the ropes of the trade as you grow. Once you have your people growing your food, all that you will need is a 'farm mother', much like a 'class mother', who volunteers to oversee the work and makes regular visits to the farm and interacts with the 'faculty' or farmers. And farm mother can be of either gender, okay?

If you own a farm already, congrats, you know what I'm talking about.

I am not asking you to store for an entire year, I know we mostly have space for about two to three months. But we can start planning for food like the way we plan for tax, reviewing it every quarter, four times a year. Basically we have to stay much more involved with food than the few minutes it's on our plate so that it actually enriches and nourishes our being. To look fresh, energetic and glowing, you should eat food that's fresh, energetic and glowing.

Btw, look at women in villages, they spend a lot of time with their food right from tilling the land, sowing seeds, cutting the crop, cleaning it, carrying it home, storing it, cooking, eating and relishing it. Who has a sexier figure, a more erect spine and an ageless face? The rural woman or the urban city chick?

Sansar sansar jasa tave chula vara, adhi hataa la chatke tevha milate bhakara — it's a popular Marathi film song picturised on women grinding grain over two stone wheels as they bend, whirl, push and pull to crush the rough grain into a powder that can then be made into a dough, rolled into a chapatti or a bhakri and then put on a tava over a chula for consumption. So the women sing, oh our life or this sansar or world is like the tava on the earthen chula: you will first burn your fingers before you can eat the bhakri or go through hardships before you can bear the fruit of your effort. So how far are you willing to go to get that fab body? All the way to the fields? If not, at least work at reducing the food miles.

How far will you go?

Here's one of my favourite stories that a client from Surat shared. One of his friends (yup, diamond merchant by profession) owns a farm on which he grows lots of local fruits and vegetables. The vegetables from his farm are especially yummy, and he is really keen that his brother, who lives in Mumbai, not miss out on them. So early every morning (yes, every single day), one of his men goes to the farm, picks up some fresh vegetables, puts them in a basket, goes to Surat station and puts the basket under a seat in one of the superfast trains. He then sms-es the seat number to the man in Mumbai, someone is sent to pick it up from Mumbai Central, it enters bhabi's kitchen, brother's plate and eventually his stomach. Nine times out of ten, he is able to get the vegetable basket, once in a while some passenger on the train gets lucky!

4. Beyond calories

I felt I had walked endlessly by the Pin river after crossing the Bhabha pass at 4900 meters. Tired, dazed and out of breath, I kept moving my legs and finally by evening I'd reached a bridge across which sat the village of Mudh. Anatomically it looks like a vagina, is what I thought to myself. It's a village with pinkish red and white homes fed by streams from two sides and it sits in the V shape in between. Awesome, I thought.

As I negotiated with my lungs and my heart started feeling light and nice, my eyes caught sight of women and children in fields where peas were being grown. The women walked up to the trail (Spitians are super friendly), bringing with them a handful of peas for me. I was more than happy to eat something so I peeled a pod, admiring how refreshingly green the peas and the peel looked (they always look tired, patchy, almost greyish in Mumbai markets). I popped the peas in my mouth — Ah, god, sweeter than sugar, I could feel fatigue vanishing from my legs and mind. 'Now eat the peel,' said the lady.

What? I may look like a monkey but I am not one, I wanted to say, but I don't take panga with locals, especially when they are in a group. So I obediently put the peel in my mouth. *Kaaraak,* it broke between my teeth and its juice sprayed across my palette and I heard myself go, Hmmm, wow! (The only expression I'd said aloud since crossing the pass.) The women giggled. You must always eat the peel, the oldest amongst them said. Good for your skin. Wow! I didn't want to tell her what happens to peas back home so I can't follow her advice as much as I believed her and would want to recreate my HMMM experience.

But why am I telling you this? Because food is not about numbers or, more specifically, calories. It's about feelings, emotion, romance, enriching and rewarding and central to human existence. It's high time we think nutrients (and our emotions while eating and the farming community's while growing, not to mention our cook's while cooking) and not calories. So this lamba chauda story is to tell you that every time somebody dismisses peas as a 'high calorie' veggie, I feel heartbroken, or rather, devastated. Peas are rich in potassium (something that could rid you of chronic bloating), vitamins B1, B2, B3 (great for when you feel tired), A, C, K and E, apart from calcium, selenium, iron, and zinc, enzymes, natural sugars, fibres. So much goodness all dismissed because it's 'badnaam' thanks to calories.

Sodium-potassium pump

During my treks with 'Connect with Himalaya', I am often amazed at how GP is much faster and 'luckier' than I am when it comes to spotting wildlife. 'The key is to look at the right places,' he explained when he sensed my envy. 'What's a "right place",' I asked, irritated. 'Dry streams, the animals often come to dry streams to lick the salt and mineral deposits off the river bed,' he explained. We are all wired to pick up and look for salt, specifically for sodium, because we are supposed to get adequate amounts of potassium from the food we eat. Yes, I am talking about the **sodium-potassium pump**. Potassium is part of what is called as intracellular or inside the cell fluid; sodium is a part of the extracellular fluid or the fluid that is outside the cells. How well our cells absorb nutrients from the blood stream, throw out waste, respond and send nerve impulses, in fact every minute function that our cells carry out depends on whether they have the right amount of sodium outside and potassium inside. Together, the sodium and potassium make the electrochemical impulse, or current-making movement inside and outside the cell, smooth and easy, in fact, possible.

Our diets, which are getting increasingly high in sodium thanks to the consumption of processed foods, fast foods and take-aways, are proving to be a big challenge to our delicately maintained Na-K pump. Add to that the fact that we are getting increasingly less fresh food, farming practices have changed and fertiliser use is higher than ever, all of which depletes the potassium stores in our body. Now when sodium increases and potassium drops, the sodium forces its way inside the cell and from there on starts the slow death of our cells because of impaired absorption of nutrients and inability to throw out waste products. Bloating or swelling is the first visible sign of this disturbed electro-chemical balance. So the next time you call for food from outside, eat too late, open a packet of diet chakli/chips, and on the other hand avoid eating 'fattening' bananas, potatoes, etc., spare a thought for the Na-K pump and the impending slow death of cells.

Nutrients

So this is where you should use buddhi, intuition and intelligence the next time somebody calls our nutrient-rich peas, carrots, potatoes, suran, sweet potato, beetroot, mangoes, rice, seetaphal, banana, chickoo, etc. 'high calorie. Please dimaag lagao; in Marathi there's a term for this — akal ghan takli ka? (loosely translated to 'have you mortgaged your brains?', used when you can't fathom really, really BASIC ideas).

You know this math? 1g carb = 4 calories, 1g protein = 4 calories, 1g of fat = 9 calories. Now if food, naturally existing in nature, is 'calorie-rich', what does it mean? That it's NUTRIENT-RICH! Oh, I have to stop screaming and stop being rude. So sorry for lacking the tact to say it in a more appropriate manner — but you are saying NO to nutrients. Food that exists in its pure form in nature on trees, grass, shrubs, creepers, etc. as a fruit, vegetable, grain, pulse is not 'fattening'. The calories are coming from the nutrients — carbs, protein, fat (usually a really small contribution) — and we need all these in our body to assimilate all the micro-nutrients like vitamins and minerals. Without adequate nutrients — the whole lot of them: carbs, protein, fat, vitamins, minerals, water, fibre — our body would never be able to enjoy optimum health, fitness or wellness. When a sense of well-being is lacking, you don't *feel* beautiful. Instead, you constantly feel inadequate.

So use your brains: if you're messing around with your fruits, vegetables, grains and processing them to a point where they've lost their nutrients and fibres, like turning them into a pulp, pickle, jam, biscuit, pastry, fruit cake, juice or frying them into chips, then yes, you're adding to the calories and removing nutrients. Avoid this messing with your food in the name of 'convenience', 'handy', 'quick snack', and to avoid calories. Calories are a good thing, trust me. On the one hand you want to look fresh and feel energetic, and on the other you want to avoid calories. **Every time you say no to calories, you say no to energy.** Energy and calories are the exact same thing. If output (body) has to be energetic, then the input (food) has to have calories. Annamaya kosha — the body is made of food. If your food is frozen, preserved, heavy on preservatives, overcooked or stale, what is your body going to look like? Anybody wants to take a wild guess?

Are you avoiding calories? Is this what your diet plan looks like?

Cereal + low fat milk
Juice
Salad with whole wheat toast
Fruit
Dry bhel or mumra
Fibre-added roti and boiled vegetables

God! Your body is going to look like it's in mourning. The cereal is rich in preservatives and sodium and perhaps also emulsifiers and permitted additives; the milk is stripped of its main nutrient, the essential fat; the juice is coloured water, stripped of fibre; the salad's been cut god knows when, and god forbid if you added low-fat dressing to give your body its daily quota of preservatives and salt; the whole wheat loaf has a shelf-life higher than chapatti so you know what *that* means; the fruit, well, what are you thinking? The body needs proper carbs, protein, fat to assimilate anything from the fruit. The dry bhel is an atyachar on your palate so the enzymes won't be interested and optimum digestion itself will not take place. The fibre 'added' to the roti is only going to 'add' to your body's woes of absorbing calcium and iron. Wow! No wonder you don't lose fat on a diet like this (weight you could lose, and with it your charm, energy and sleep).

My name is carb and I am not fattening

Inspired entirely by *My Name is Khan* (and I am not a terrorist). When you take out of a potato, banana, rice, wheat (also seetaphal, chickoo, mango, grapes) what makes them nutritious and energy-giving and turn them into items that are filled with preservatives, additives, permitted colourings, emulsifiers, salts and, worse, the added 'healthy' fibre, calcium, iron, etc., they no longer remain usable for the body.

Just like terror has no colour or religion, junk has no health or nutritional value.

Actually, adding 'health' or 'religion' to junk may sell it better and even find credibility with the gullible, but does it help add to physical, emotional, mental, spiritual well-being? No, it erodes it in a cruel manner, bringing disrepute to the entire 'food group' or 'community', spreads fear and makes our lives dull, limited and boring. Think about how the roti and rice feel when you leave it out of your life, thinking that they are harmful, and choose to eat only salad or soup or sabzi + dal? Devastated, misunderstood and let down, you bet.

So when you remove fibre, niacin and vitamin B, zinc, selenium and a host of other vitamins, minerals and enzymes from carbs, it no longer remains a carb, it simply turns to junk. Is junk fattening? Yes. Can you turn carb to junk? Yes, by removing all that makes it a carb. You could apply the same process to protein, fat, water and turn them to junk too. (Water to cola, meat to sausage, white butter to yellow butter or margarine.) Just because they do it primarily with carbs, it hasn't earned them that label yet. And avoiding carbs is leading to lifestyle disorders, unstable blood sugars, constipation, sleepless nights, dull skin — the list is endless. Junk is junk, avoid it but don't badnaamofy carbs, at least not in our country where they are an integral part of our culture and cuisine.

Cooking traditions

And that brings me to another point: our traditional recipes and cooking. What's this whole fuss about boiled veggies and steamed veggies? What's so wrong with the tadka? The Indian style of cooking liberally uses hing, turmeric, jeera, sesame, curry leaves, green chillies and many other spices, condiments and herbs to give a dish its distinct flavour, aroma and taste. Now ask Tarla Dalal or Sanjeev Kapoor and they will tell you that food and the way you cook is an expression of divinity itself. It's an underrated art, and our own distinct style of cooking is a legacy worth preserving, documenting and practising.

Every region in our diverse country has its own distinct style of cooking. A north Indian's dal is different from a south Indian's, which differs from the Marathi dal and that of the Rajasthani and that of the Assamese. Now within this too, every community, caste, tribe, village will have its own 'secret' ingredient and recipe. It's just too bad that we have failed to package and market it as exotic, magical or 'fat-burning'. But don't let that take away from the fact that it actually is exotic, magical and fat-burning. Vir Sanghvi (I think he has brilliant insights on food, cooking, restaurants and the art of eating; plus, he looks good) wrote an article on how we are losing our local cuisine to global cuisine. Learning from the rest of the globe is always a good thing; adopting things which appeal to you is great; letting go of what you already have and what is useful (though not valued) is NOT.

This art of knowing exactly when to add the spices to the oil, or the science of how long you should heat the oil, or whether you put the hing first or the haldi is worth the effort because it aids digestion, assimilation, excretion, yes, but it also has anti-ageing, memory-sharpening, muscle-toning, fat-reducing and even cancer-preventing properties. But we will let go of this because we want to avoid calories or think yummy = fattening, yucky = lose weight, get thin quickly. Now you just boil the vegetable, or make it into a sabzi but don't add the tadka, and eat it virtuously. Do you get all the fat-burning, anti-ageing, digestion-aiding, yummy-tasting and therapeutic properties of tazaa ghar ka khana? No, you get grief. So learn to enjoy life by learning to enjoy food. (Please don't confuse 'enjoy' with 'greed', dabaoing or sensory overload associated with stuffing your mouth.)

Filtered oil

So what about oils and frying — is that not 'fattening'? Not if you apply the three strategies mentioned above: use local oil, respect the rule of Uno (know where to stop), and involve yourself a bit in how your oil was made. We Indians use a lot of groundnut oil, ghee and in some regions sesame, mustard and coconut oil. Now here's the thing, when you buy oil, look for the word 'filtered'. Filtered oil involves a process where the seed from which the oil is extracted is subjected to lower temperatures than 'refined' oils. So what does that mean for us? Lower temperature means less damage to the fat-soluble vitamins like A, D, E (rich in antioxidant properties), less damage to the molecular structure of fatty acid bonds in the seed (so more heart-protecting properties) and the need to use good quality seeds because of the smell and because impurities will not be destroyed at low temperatures (better seed = better aroma, flavour while cooking).

So are we using filtered oil made from our traditional methods, which use a wooden ghana or vessel and low temperatures? Not really. Two main contributing reasons for this: 1) They are not sold as 'heart-protecting and antioxidant rich', will retain some colour (often and wrongly associated with cheap or for 'poor people'), are not available in fancy bottles — basically poor packaging and marketing and 2) The high costs involved in making oils the traditional way as the seeds won't give out all their oil.

The economical way of making oil involves using solvents, high temperatures and technology to extract every little bit of oil that can be squeezed from the seed. And because the squeezing is so complete, you can use a lower grade of seed. Now you have a really 'cheap' oil, or better yield (more oil extracted per seed). The fancy bottles that you find in supermarkets with 'added antioxidants and vitamins' (they have to, their processes are killing the naturally existing bonds and antioxidants, even changing the molecular structure of bonds within the fatty acids by a process called 'polymerisation' which can be potentially damaging to the heart) are mostly the refined oils. They also have tons of money to market and grab your 'mind space' as heart-protecting oils. This is called 'yeda banke pedha khaneka', Mumbaiya for pretentious attitude. So people, **use 'filtered' or 'cold-pressed' or 'virgin' oils to get the maximum nutrients from your oil.** Don't let them go home with money earned from your ignorance.

Brown or white?

Shift to brown rice — heard that dictum before? Okay, chew on this: white rice, where we pound the rice to remove its outer covering, is not at all bad, in fact it's great. The bad thing is when we mindlessly decide if one thing is good for us and that if we do it a lot, it becomes only better. We do that with rice so often now.

Every rice season, as we joined our ajoba (paternal grandfather) in our farm in Sonave (outside Mumbai), we would see women pounding, cleaning, shifting rice endlessly from sunrise to sunset. Pounding rice removes the outer layer of the rice, and with it part of the fibre and vitamin B too. Is fibre and vitamin B good for you? Absolutely. So why are they doing it? To remove the husk and bran, the outer part of the rice; but the protein, vitamin B and fibre *inside* the grain is still retained.

In fact, the protein in white rice is absorbed much better by your body than that in brown rice. It is also way easier to cook and digest white rice as compared to brown rice. Anywhere in India, when you are sick and down, what are you given? Khichdi. And khichdi has white rice, sweeties: it's easy to digest, easy to absorb, easy to assimilate proteins from and easier on your excretory system too. Ayurveda uses rice-based diets in treating various imbalances in the body. If rice that's devoid of its husk and bran is as 'fattening' as it's made out to be, all of our coastal belt would be floating in their backwaters (fat floats), but are they?

To get the best of both the worlds, polish your rice but not to the extent that it emits blinding whiteness. Remove the outer bran but allow the rice grain to show off its brown/red strains (this is what I refer to as brown rice, not the wrongly understood one with the husk and bran intact). No, don't worry, this won't compromise on the taste, and yes, you can totally eat your basmati with the red/brown strains too. This is exactly how the farming community of India eats their rice. Ever checked out their sizzling waists and six packs?

PS: Also, as India is dominantly vegetarian, getting proteins from rice, especially the essential amino acid methionine, branched chain amino acids and the conditionally essential (becomes essential under conditions of stress) amino acid tyrosine is crucial for us. So if you are vegetarian, stop fussing over rice all the more, just eat it.

PPS: You can eat rice even if you are diabetic. Chill. You need those proteins too.

Sweet visa

And what about sweets and desserts, won't they make us fat? No, not if you apply all strategies above, and then apply what I call as the rule of 'visa'. Stood in big queues for your US visa only to have it rejected by a rude officer? Then you know what I'm talking about. Big and strong nations don't hand out visas to all and sundry. They make their own evaluations (based on their own logic) and make decisions about who they consider 'worthy' of entry into their country. A weak nation, however, hands out visas quite liberally. So when it comes to your stomach, make it like a super-power nation, which decides not just the number of visas, let's say H1 visas, that will be handed out every year, but also who it will be handed out to. So the number of times you eat a dessert in the year should be strictly controlled like the H1 visa. If you've allotted thirty-six, twelve, fifty-two, whatever number (once a month, twice a month, and a day each of Diwali + one for birthday, anniversary, grandpa's eightieth whatever — up to you to decide), get prudent with it and hand it over to only 'worthy' occasions. So bad mood and feel like a pastry won't count as worthy, but 'first salary' or anything that's meaningful in your life gets the visa. Once you exhaust your allotted number you are not allowed to allot more visas. Also if you hand it over to 'unworthy' situations, it's your fault. See, the American embassy will take your papers almost two months prior to your interview. Take a leaf out of their book and take applications well in advance so that you can make thoughtful decisions on giving your 'sweet visa' to the right situation.

So as long as we eat according to the four principles and learn to apply the nutrition strategies, we don't need to kick ourselves over the occasional sweet or fried item. It's really not going to make us fat or destroy our diet; it is in fact accepted as part of our diet.

II

Exercise Strategies

If you have an an ass, move it.

–Anonymous (or maybe I said it in one of my bright moments)

What would you do if you were made prime minister for a day? 'I will build a huge sports complex,' she said, and there Madhu Sapre lost her chance to become Miss Universe in 1992. She was the front runner to win the crown, and she almost did, till she displayed her 'insensitivity' and actually said in so many words that she would build a sports complex. Here was a good-looking woman from a poor country like India: shouldn't she care about poverty, children and world peace? 'But then they asked us to speak straight from the heart (and not be politically correct), and in a year what can one do about poverty (anybody who comes from a poor country knows that), but a sports complex is doable and it can make the poor feel at par with the rich,' reasoned Madhu later. Sounds reasonable, right? But the bias against women and what they are supposed to feel sympathy for is universal, as universal as the concept of peace, love, harmony. Women constantly carry this burden of the assumption that we're supposed to put children, education, poverty, home, peace, etc. over our own health, fitness, wellness. The next time you feel that stabbing guilt when you make your way to the gym, reason with yourself: if I have to work at my best, mother at my best, play all the multiple roles I have chosen for myself with ease and without being tired and irritated, then I must invest my time wisely and spend time strengthening and nurturing my physical body.

Now I do know that most women will be left with very little time to themselves and then, of course, there are simply too many 'valid reasons' (read excuses) as to why we must postpone exercising to tomorrow/Monday/next month/next year and sometime after little Babloo starts going to school or maybe after he passes his 10th Std or whatever.

But I can't emphasise enough the need to stay physically fit and to indulge in regular, hardcore exercise. Women are exposed to many biologically challenging events: regular menstrual cycles, childbearing, rearing, nursing, and then sociological reasons like moving with the family and husband (often without having a say in the matter), learning to make compromises on every front (and without complaints), etc. We should be working out and keeping fit out of biological necessity and not out of some pressure to stay or look thin. However, it's often us women who, as little girls, will give up on exercising or simply running around the grounds, jumping, hanging on branches, twisting, shoving, pulling, pushing basically anything 'hardcore' (boyish/manly) the minute we reach puberty, which is such a shame, really! The minute girls in my building hit 7th-8th Std, they just start standing around in packs, and at the most do rounds of the building.

I think that's why Madhu Sapre wanted a sports complex. As an athlete, she understood the downside of the lack of facilities. Think about it, if you have parents paying for fancy club memberships, even then you have to rise above social conventions of what is considered 'boyish', or more 'important' (such as 10th/12th Std exams) and continue playing your sport. If your parents are not rich enough to buy memberships, what do you do, roam around the building or your mohalla? Waiting to grow up to buy a membership is one option. You could rise above the social conventions of what is considered more important at your age (probably marriage/giving birth, etc.) and pursue a sport then. But the thing is, if you've been an active and fit teenager, then, a) you don't get fat during your shaadi/work/mothering periods and b) even if you do, your chances of getting back in shape and quickly are sky high.

We all have to realise that it is as important for our girls, daughters, mothers, sisters, aunts, grandmothers to indulge in hardcore physical activity and sports, as it is for us to have womankind educated, literate and encouraged to pursue higher education. (You know how some families, specially the fathers-in-law, will khao bhav and tell everybody who is willing to listen that they insisted that the bahu finish her education and did everything to ensure that she can pursue it post marriage without any disturbance, etc.? They need to talk about our fitness in the exact same vein. 'I told my bahu, no giving up on your game/gym/morning run/yoga.' Now I would give a million dollars to hear that [earn and give, of course ☺].)

Now I guess we all know how education affects and improves not just the life of the woman directly, but also that of her children, family, community or world at large. The exact same reasons are valid for women to remain physically fit. It's the physically fit who will be the leaders, game changers, thinkers, scientists, path-breakers. Yoga, running, weight-training, swimming, playing a game, dancing, group exercises — everything works (provided it fulfils the criteria listed further ahead in the section).

Equal opportunity

Invariably on our treks, after lunch, the boys will suggest playing a sport, usually cricket. They will draw great pleasure from making bats out of a log of wood and making stumps out of some branches, hunt for a ball and have a blast playing. The girls (mostly women who are quite in shape) will only look on enviously. Most of these women are independent, as competent, or better than the men in their chosen fields, and invariably shouldering much more responsibility than the men in their lives. But when it comes to outdoor games, women have had to face the gross injustice of a lack of equal opportunity. Boys continue playing through their high school, into college, etc., and at the most give up because of 'work hours'. Sadly, women give up playing sometime in high school, and then their 'work life' extends itself way beyond office hours. I know our parents (especially mothers) will be disturbed/lecture us if we don't study hard in school, worry about our dark future and difficult life. What is their response if we don't play hardcore during these years? How many mothers have been genuinely upset that their girls are no longer playing a sport? Are they even aware of the dangers looming in their girls' futures if they don't play? They are darker than not getting admission in a specific college for a specific course. These dangers will prevent the girls from enjoying life to its optimum and, worst case scenario, could lead to fatal conditions. Rise and shine mothers, it's up to you — push your girls hard, push them to exercise, push them towards physical learning and push by setting a fine example.

> The funny part is women trek just as well as the men, so physical fitness is not really the issue, the issue is deeper — that of discrimination. Since a trek is a space for equal opportunity, both genders do well and the ability to enjoy it to the fullest is not hindered by discrimination.

Let's look at some crucial concepts of exercise:

1. Kinesthetic intelligence
2. Five pillars of fitness
3. The principles of exercising right

1. Kinesthetic intelligence

When an old aunt slips in the bathroom, she falls and in all probability suffers a fracture and has to be helped out of the bathroom. When a young child slips in the bathroom, she gets joy out of the feeling of sliding on the slippery wet bathroom floor. She probably doesn't crash down to the floor, but even if she does, she almost never suffers a fracture, much less needs any rescue effort. The act of falling is the same, the same bathroom, the same degree of wetness, slipperiness, etc., then why does the aunt suffer a fracture and the child only enjoy the feeling of falling? The answer is kinesthetic intelligence: the child has the body intelligence to know which muscles to contract, which ones to relax, which joint to flex, which one to extend, to prevent the fall; and if she does fall, she has the intelligence to know how to take it while minimising the load or weight on her joints. So even before she falls, she stands up. If you have seen Jonty Rhodes fielding at the point, then you know what I am talking about. On more than one occasion it seems like he is going to crash into the stumps or break one of his bones or at least strain, sprain or pull a muscle. No, sorry, his kinesthetic intelligence is just sky-high. My favourite sports picture is of Jonty Rhodes parallel to the floor at the height of the stumps, with his arm extended and the ball hitting the bails; the caption reads: It's a plane, it's a bird, it's JONTY RHODES!

Okay, okay, I know you have no plans of being a cricketer and much less Jonty Rhodes, but if you want to look sexy, toned, youthful and energetic, and not suffer fractures in your old age because of falls, or a backache because of a long flight, or cramps in the calf after a day of wearing stilettos, then you need to pay attention to kinesthetic intelligence. And for this, just like you go to school sincerely and dedicatedly without missing it for a day, you have to regularly play, work out, dance, practise martial arts — basically anything that employs the body, its nerves, joints, muscles, bones, organs, etc. Use your body and use it regularly to keep it in great shape. To give another example, remember how about nine-ten years ago, in the good old days, each one of us could remember at least ten phone numbers by heart? Now with mobile phones and their memories, we don't even remember our partner's, parent's or office phone number. Use it or lose it.

2. Five pillars of fitness

Let's assume that there is a workout school out there that you could attend. You'd be taught five main subjects: cardio-respiratory fitness, muscular endurance, muscular strength, flexibility and body composition. You cannot do any justice to the time spent working out or the calories burnt if they do not lead to any kind of progress or learning in these five core areas of fitness.

Cardio respiratory fitness: Ability of the heart and lungs (also called as cardio-pulmonary fitness) to deliver oxygen and nutrients to working cells or muscles which are demanding them. Let's say you're climbing stairs: your leg muscles will demand more blood supply, oxygen and nutrient delivery, and will need to remove or recycle waste products (like lactic acid).

Muscular strength: The greatest amount of force (maximal effort) that a muscle or a group of muscles can exert at one time. Ever watched a cop lagao a lafa? That's muscular strength. Or when Sunny Deol says, 'Yeh dhai kilo ka haath jab padta hai to aadmi uthta nahi, uth jata hai'. The technical term in exercise physiology is 'one rep max' but apna Bollywood describes it better.

Muscular endurance: The ability of a muscle or a group of muscles to perform repeated activity over a period of time. For example, if you're moving furniture or if you're making laddoos, then you'll be using your muscular endurance.

Flexibility: Ability of the joints to move through their full range of motion (ROM). For example, a bowler would move her arm through a full range of motion of her shoulder before the delivery.

Body composition: This refers to the fat mass that you carry as compared to the total body mass you have. For women this should be twenty-five per cent or under. So even if you weigh a hundred kilos, not more than twenty-five kilos should come from fat. When women say they want to look toned and not flabby, they actually mean that they would like to reduce the fat mass and increase their lean mass (bone and muscle).

Now, the moral of the story is when you make improvements on the first four parameters of fitness, it results in an improvement (lowering fat mass) in the fifth parameter, that of body composition. Learning these 'subjects' or making improvements on these fitness parameters leads to an improvement in overall health, sense of well-being, sharpens your kinesthetic intelligence and, ya, improves your appearance as well. It also leads to perfect harmony in our hormones, stable moods and puts the mind into 'feel good' mode, unlike the high-strung or run-down state of mind that most weight loss plans lead to.

One of the reasons why I call the book 'weight loss tamasha' is exactly this. **No one seems to talk about getting fitter, sharpening the kinesthetic intelligence, improving quality of life, increasing the well-being quotient, etc**. All that we seem to care about is losing inches and getting that needle on the weighing scale to move down. Any weight loss or inch loss achieved without an improvement on the five fitness parameters above is a tamasha, a joke, cheating, a criminal waste of time, money and resources. What are we thinking when we buy into those 'two months, five kilos' (buy fifteen kilos and get three kilos free for any family member — my favourite ad), 'seven sessions, nine kilos' guarantees, one week 'detox' before shaadi, etc.? If we don't think about asking questions like, will it make my knees stronger, bones denser, skin smoother, hair thicker, mind calmer, hunger signals sharper, etc., then we deserve the diets we get, pretty much like we deserve the politicians we get because we don't ask them the right questions or give a damn for accountability (other than living room conversations of course).

So let's understand this well. Weight loss is a byproduct (but not essential) of an improvement in body composition, which in turn is an essential by-product of improvement in the first four parameters of fitness. If you want to save your skin literally (sagging, wrinkles) and figuratively, then you must opt for fitness and weight loss programmes that are not sold or popular for 'weight loss'. Samjha? Don't buy into programmes that say 'pay x and lose y kilos'. Also, don't go under the knife to lose weight. Simply because weight lost at the cost of a decrease in all five core fitness parameters (which is what most 'diets', 'procedures', 'surgeries', 'toning tables', 'techniques', 'herbal or ayurvedic pill/potions' do), is simply worthless.

And no, these five areas of fitness are not meant only for athletes or sports persons, they are meant for people like you and me, the ones who do a lot of sitting around and lead sedentary lifestyles. Athletes or sportspersons need these five core areas and then build on other parameters specific to their sport, like agility, power, speed, hand-eye coordination, etc. Why am I telling you all this? Because I want to make sure that you don't tell yourself that this is for sports people/size zero/youngsters/celebs, etc. **This is for all of us and we can improve at any age, at any weight.** These are the very basic foundations of nurturing the physical body to use it like a vehicle fit to pursue higher goals of human life (the Vedic tradition, in fact all religious traditions adhere to this view). No higher purpose can be achieved when you lose those two or twenty kilos or fit into a size six or whatever, but it can be when you have enough energy and enthusiasm left at the end of your day. Incidentally, this is also how exercise science describes physical fitness: to go through day-to-day activities without feeling unduly tired and to have enough energy left to tackle emergencies, pursue hobbies, exercise or higher spiritual goals.

Learn to take time off

I had signed up for an intensive yoga course at my ashram in Netala. Just six days into the course, the asana, pranayama and bandha practice three times a day, and waking up at unusually early hours, left me feeling sick, tired and feverish. On the seventh day, I skipped the early morning prayer and chanting session and lay in bed, sleeping. By 6.30 a.m., my roomies returned to the dorm to pick up their mats and stuff for the asana practice that would start by 7 a.m. Startled, I got up feeling guilty about missing the early morning class and miserable about not having enough self-discipline. I gave myself a pep talk on why I was there and how I had to optimise my time and learn everything that I could in these fifteen days and blah blah. Fully charged now, I got dressed, rolled up my mat, carried my notebook and braved my way to the asana hall by the Bhagirathi river. 'Where are you going Rujuta?' asked my teacher, Swami Govindananda, blocking my way at the entrance of the hall. 'To the class, Swamiji,' I replied, with a sense of pride and dignity. 'With fever?' he asked. 'Yes, I already missed the morning class and can't miss more, I am here to learn.' 'Good then learn this, go back to your dorm.' I thought the swamiji would be proud of me for having the courage to fulfil my 'responsibility or obligation' to attend morning practice. I also thought he would be disappointed/upset with me for sleeping in late during a course. Instead here he was, blocking my way to the entrance hall and not a wee bit angry. Dejected and miserable I walked back to the dorm. I just couldn't figure out why he was acting the way he was. He followed me and said, 'Come let's sit in the garden, and bring your shawl.' I obeyed. 'Swamiji, why?' I asked when I was in the garden, watching my course-mates getting into serious asana practice while I sat twiddling my thumbs and swinging my legs aimlessly. 'Because you have a fever, it's your body's way of saying "no asana practice today".' 'That's it?' I asked rudely, feeling let down by my body. 'So I go through nine hours of practice for six days and on the seventh day I have fever? I am really so disappointed with my body.' 'Why? You should be grateful to her. Grateful that she is kind enough to tell you what her limits are. Good that you get fever, or else you will not learn to respect the body's limitations and even less learn how to overcome them.

'So take the day off, week off, whatever time the body needs to adapt and don't work against your body, work with her. She does whatever you want from her. Do you ever do a nine-hour practice in Mumbai?' 'No, not even ninety minutes.' 'Then, first thank the body that whenever you bring up a nine-hour practice, for six days she can keep up with the demand and only asks for a day's rest.

'Maybe this time your lesson here is this — learning to be grateful to your body for showing you her limits, being happy with yourself that you have the courage to push your body to the limits, and more importantly to stop at the first sign or demand to slow down. This is the only way both you and your body can learn.' My disappointment was replaced with gratefulness and once more I thought to myself how unlimited access to committed and experienced teachers is so important. No wonder the gurukul system produced finer students and individuals compared to our 7 a.m. to 2 p.m. or noon to 6 p.m. schools.

The day before, I had 'read' that when the body is tired, has fever for example, there should be no asana practice, according to the Hatha yoga pradipika. It could harm you and weaken your nervous system. But had I learnt to bring that into practice? No, not until the morning I woke up sick.

So why am I telling you all this? Because it really makes sense to not work out when you are tired mentally or physically and it makes no sense to push yourself when all you should do is skip and chill.

3. The principles of exercise

To make the most improvement in these five areas, we need to follow the guidelines or principles of exercise. These are rules that will make your exercise routine effective, i.e., will enable you to burn fat during and after exercise and ensure progress, learning and sharpening of your kinesthetic intelligence.

i. Progressive overload principle, often called the mother of all training or exercise principles. This means that the stress or stimuli that you put your body through during training should be greater than what you normally encounter in your day-to-day activities and should increase in an incremental order.

This is one reason why 'walking' doesn't qualify as exercise. You walk from your bed to the bathroom or from your car to the lift. So when you go for a 'walk', you are not exactly overloading the system and therefore the benefits that you achieve on your five core fitness parameters are limited. Now read the name of the principle again: PROGRESSIVE overload principle. This means that even if you choose to walk as a means of exercise, then you must progressively learn to do more during your walk. For example, run for some time in between the walk, or try walking the same distance in less time.

ii. Specific Adaptation to Imposed Demands (SAID). A crucial principle to your fitness routine, this one is based on the most basic ability in us humans — the ability to adapt. Simply put, it means that our body and all its systems (nervous system, our circulatory system, cardiopulmonary system, skeletal system, basically every system and metabolic pathway) adapt to the specific demands or stresses that we put on them. Ever wondered why you only find certain species of animals in certain latitudes on Earth, but humans can live anywhere from the North Pole to the South Pole? SAID is at work, humans adapt.

So a Ladakhi would have a system adapted and therefore 'suitable' to altitude, while a Keralite will have a system that can dissipate heat better and help her deal with humidity and heat. It also means that the Keralite will get mountain sickness in Ladakh and a Ladakhi will get sea sickness in Kerala, ha ha ha, kya PJ mara hai!

Coming back to what we are really talking about. Basically, what this means is that, when you 'warm up' on the treadmill before a resistance or weight-training session, you falter on the SAID principle and will expose your body to injuries. To help your body perform better at resistance or weight-training, your warm-up should consist of weight- or resistance-training but at a lower intensity than your main workout. So if your 'main set' is 10 lbs for 15 reps, then the warm-up can be 5 lbs for 5 reps. It also means that your warm-up should be specific to the muscles used during the workout. If you're training your back, the warm-up should be for the back and not for the chest, get it?

The progressive overload comes before SAID, because without overload, adaptation cannot take place. It also means that if the overload is too little or too much, then injury, boredom or a plateau effect occurs.

iii. Recovery. This comes after SAID, because whether or not you will adapt depends entirely on whether or not you will recover. I hope you're getting this: first you must choose the right stimuli (exercise) to overload (not more, not less) then you must recover from this stimuli to allow adaptation to occur. When recovery is compromised, adaptation doesn't occur; it means you don't make progress on the five core areas and therefore you are wasting your time burning those precious calories. Good recovery means good nutrition + hydration + sleep. So if you really want that fab body, eat right, drink right, sleep right. No shortcuts. This is also why I often say that eating right and working out are like two sides of the same coin. Only exercise, and being careless about eating right = lack of recovery = zero or at best limited result = frustration. Eating right but not working out = no overload = zero or limited result = frustration.

iv. Regularity. Ha, ha, this is my personal favourite. The use it or lose it funda is based on this. The SAID principle leads to us having something called as 'muscle memory', much like brain memory. So if you are not regular with your workouts, you will go through something called as 'detraining' or 'de-conditioning'. Essentially, it means that your body will lose its kinesthetic intelligence and will get poorer at the five core areas of fitness. Gosh! Sounds like a nightmare. So if you wanna look sharp, toned, sexy, then train (exercise) with regularity. Read *regularity*, and not *daily*. Just ensure that you use all the previous three principles first to get the max out of your workout. Let me explain. You walk daily but don't care for overload = no improvement in the fitness parameters = kya time ka khoti! You train hard, almost kill yourself in the gym and then eat late night and don't sleep on time, so no recovery = no improvement on the fitness parameters = aunty, sudhar jao!

God, digressing again. I was making the point of muscle memory. This refers to nerves per unit of muscle fibre or the neural pathway your muscles will use to bring about an action. See, your right hand (or left, if you're a leftie) gets used frequently so you are stronger, sharper or can write with ease with that hand. The other hand doesn't get used regularly, so it is weak and can't write. Let's say you are thirty and attempting to write a three-hour paper when the last time you took an exam like that was when you were fifteen. Now, when you begin writing, the right hand will hurt at first but will slowly refresh its memory of writing exams and will eventually write like a pro. But the left hand still won't be able to write because it lacks the 'memory'.

Or let's say you were training regularly, then shaadi, baccha-kachha and it's been ten years since you exercised, but within weeks of starting to exercise again your body will ignite its muscle memory and bring your fitness parameters to where you last left them.

All in all, people with accumulated fitness or those who have a history of keeping fit will find it easier to make gains on the core fitness parameters when they start using the principles above. So women, don't let your past get in the way of your present and say, 'I used to be so fit and now look at me'. Simply start and in no time you will be back to your original fitness levels.

Word of caution: detraining can occur in about three weeks, so don't go without exercise for over three weeks, okay? It's very expensive metabolically for your body to maintain 'conditioning' or high levels of core fitness parameters, so if your body doesn't get the right stimuli to maintain it, it will bring the cost down and lower its metabolic spending. Bole ga toh, 'conditioning' means your first four core fitness parameters are well developed so your body will be leaner and fitter, carrying more muscle as compared to the fat it carries. Muscle is metabolically active tissue, it forces the body to burn fat to maintain itself, so if the muscles are not being used, the body will reduce spending on its fat tissue and detrain or lose the muscle tissue. Getting it? Low BMR = more body fat.

v. **Principle of balance or variation**. This simply means that the first four fitness parameters must be stimulated, adapted, recovered and trained regularly. In other words, if you only build strength and ignore flexibility or only work on cardio and ignore strength, then instead of getting fitter you will lose out on fitness and increase the chances of getting injured. Basically there are no short cuts. The next time somebody says 'just start walking' as a solution to your fitness, tell them that it won't address all the fitness parameters and therefore is not the 'best' exercise. Also, remember the next time somebody says 'use variation or you will not get results', it is coming out of a misunderstanding of the principle of variation or balance. You need to use a variety of exercises because you need to develop and stimulate various parameters of fitness. It doesn't mean a mindless switching from yoga to aerobics to weight-training. You need to build a well-rounded or complete (that which includes all the parameters) fitness programme, planned and executed based on the core training principles.

Adiponectin

Dr Len Kravtiz, an exercise physiologist, described it as a 'good guy hormone' at a fitness conference I attended in NYC. This hormone is secreted by the fat cells in the body. The leaner (lower fat weight and higher bone and muscle weight) and fitter you are, the more the adiponectin your fat cells produce. Adiponectin prevents occurrence of the metabolic syndrome that is associated with a higher risk of osteoporosis, high blood pressure, heart disease, diabetes, etc. See we need body fat; fat protects us from all the 'obesity'-related diseases by secreting the 'good guy hormone'. All we need is to support our fat cells with adequate bone and muscle tissue. Good news? Promise to stop pinching your thighs with contempt and work on improving your lifestyle instead. Want some more good news? Adiponectin also helps you reduce cellular inflammation, what we commonly refer to as 'bloating'. So just get fitter darlings.

III

Sleep strategies

Not everything that can be counted counts, and not everything that counts can be counted.

–Albert Einstein

Einstein could well have been talking about the association of body weight and sleep. Body weight and weight loss can be counted but doesn't count for much (when it comes to your health, fitness and peace), as you have by now (fingers crossed) understood, but sleep does. Sadly, sleep can't really be quantified or qualified, or at least it's complicated to do so. But you can experience and know for sure that when you don't sleep well, your recovery suffers, you wake up tired, feel bloated, lethargic and generally are like a zombie, and there go your exercise and diet plans or at least they get pushed to the next day. This is clearly the most overlooked and underappreciated aspect of 'weight loss' (fat loss, improved body composition). (Like how a housewife's contribution to running an efficient kitchen and home pushes the husband's business profits higher; you can't prove it, but you *know* there is a strong link and you wish there were a conclusive way to prove it.)

Lack of sleep, and I mean good quality sleep, will push your diet and exercise plans to the next day, therefore keeping you FAT for today, and could even lead to a host of lifestyle and metabolic disorders like PCOS, thyroid malfunction, diabetes, high blood pressure, osteoporosis, etc., basically keeping you from expressing your potential and enjoying your life to the fullest.

Overeating followed by long gaps between meals (an underlying factor in gaining body fat) is not a vicious cycle, it's a downward spiral, and lack of sleep contributes to it. When you wake up tired and groggy you need a stimulant to wake you up so you have a cup of coffee/tea, and from there on begins the atyachar on your digestive system. You lose touch with the hunger signals your body's sending you, will eat nothing for up to four hours (or more) and eventually end up gobbling every morsel that flies past you. If you decide to give in to the feeling of 'five minutes more', you end up sleeping much longer (always) and then have difficulty sleeping in the night. Staying up at night is the prequel to midnight snacking. So deviyon, waking up fresh is the only option and forms a non-negotiable Strategy 3 to lose weight.

I really can't over-emphasise the importance of a restful night; to be able to sleep at will is nothing short of a blessing. 'Gudakesh' is one of the names by which Sri Krishna calls Arjuna in the *Bhagvad Gita*. It means somebody who is so powerful that he has gained control over sleep. Arjuna could sleep (and stay awake) at will. One must not eat or sleep too much (or too little) is one of the messages of the *Gita*, and religions world over have the same message — that it is important to be disciplined about sleeping and eating if one is to enjoy and actualise the vast human potential. For now we will limit this to the human potential to lose weight.

In our 'modern' (messed up) life, human intelligence is used to create flat screen TVs which can be watched lying down, and thick curtains can be employed to block sunlight from entering your bedroom and disturbing you from the deep sleep that you invariably fall into in the early hours of the morning (between 6 and 9 o'clock). The SAID principle (see Exercise Strategies) works boss, wherever you employ it, so your body adapts to the TV, thick curtains in the bedroom and quickly gets rid of 'unwanted' (lean) tissue of the body and gets fat as a response to the sedentary lifestyle.

To reverse the damage (or adaptation), we need to undo what we have become used to by following these Sleep strategies:

1. No TV in the bedroom
2. No booze before sleeping
3. No stimulant before sunset
4. No compensation

1. No TV in the bedroom. Ya, I know you can afford a flat screen and it has BEE rating and that it is blah blah blah, but come on, it's not worth it ladies. Not when that fat pops over the sides of your jeans and right on top of your zipper. The bigger the TV, the bigger the size of your jeans; the flatter the TV, the rounder your stomach. God, I think I am a walking, talking Ramsay film, sounds like a horror story na?

Hindustani classical music is one of the things that we all will bhav maro on (specially in front of firangs or when in phoren), but will give a damn about when it comes to actually applying or practising this wisdom (yes sweety, it's wisdom not just art) in our daily lives. Music originates from the Sama ved, and in classical music certain ragas are meant to be listened to at particular times. Heard about ratri ka pehla prahar, dopahar ka doosra prahar, etc., right?

So much for the Vedic culture, sanskriti, sabhyata if we 'unwind or sleep' listening to random, loud, screeching noises from the TV. The news anchors are not talking in the sur or sargam that's recommended for 'ratri ka prahar' nor are the saas, bahus, bechari betis or akha parivaar or whatever you watch. On the one hand we would like to take digs at the Ekta Kapoor (I feel we should add 'the' before her name, she is the TV empress, easily) or find *Peepli Live* a great satire, but on the other hand we will lap up anything they dole out to us and we will do it daily. So who is the joke on? Ekta Kapoor, media, or on you, ma'am?

Watching and hearing sounds from TV robs you of restful sleep that is oh so essential for fat loss. 'Oh! I wonder how she goes to sleep every night.' If you have ever said that about somebody who's going through a rough period in her life, or has done some lafda like chori or extramarital affair, or forgotten to pick up her daughter from school one day, etc. (ya, ya, we are such judgmental bitches), then remember that lights and sounds in the night emitting from the TV, laptop, PlayStation are stressful and qualify as an offence too. Yes, you are cheating your biological clock, and if I were you and nursed dreams of fitting into a tight choli and wearing a saree three inches below my navel, arrey baapre, I wouldn't ever dare to cheat my biological clock. Here's why.

The biological clock

The biological clock (the suprachiasmatic nucleus or SCN) is a tiny little mungi-sized structure which has haathi-sized effects on weight loss. It is located in the hypothalamus region, contains over 20,000 neurons and is strategically placed at a point where it can stay in constant touch with the optic nerves. So your eyes constantly tell the SCN whether it's day or night or twilight, etc. The SCN tells all other parts of your brain including the pineal gland what to do depending on the time. So if it's evening or night, the mungi will tell the pineal gland to secrete the hormone melatonin which will induce sleep. Now if your eyes have picked up the radiation from the TV (or the laptop) then — dhan te nan — no melatonin, let's activate catecholamines instead. Catecholamines are hormones which put your body in the fight or flight mode (opposite of inducing sleep; it induces feelings of alertness — ready to kill or die) and are secreted by the adrenal glands above your kidney. This group of hormones also interferes with another hormone called leptin, which is secreted by your fat cells and decreases its levels. Leptos is Greek for 'thin', so the levels of this hormone which induces satiety (prevents overeating and keeps you thin) and asks you to stop eating, goes down and your brain asks you to eat. Think about it: late-night movie and a bucket of popcorn — is the puzzle getting solved for you? So the ghar ka equivalent of watching TV before sleeping or having it in the bedroom with the 'adjusting' husband putting on ear phones to save you from the noise and the 'stubborn' wife getting exposed only to radiation = a wife who feels 'not full or wants something meetha' after a meal or 'feels like a pastry' in the night or 'sleep walks' to the fridge in the night. God! Even writing about it makes me sick!

So you want me to say it again? **Say NO to TV in the bedroom, say YES to the saree and wear it three inches below the navel.** Ha, ha, can I get a job as a copywriter? Guess not, so I will proceed to writing the second sleep strategy.

Sleep and intuition

The Bihar School of Yoga has worked extensively on exploring 'Yog Nidra' and has used its 'magical' powers to teach math tables to sleeping children or teach yoga to jail inmates. Can you learn or awaken your intuition in your sleep? Yes, it's been proved beyond doubt that sleep improves well-being, learning abilities and memory powers. August Kekule discovered the cyclic structure of Benzene in his sleep. Till he slept over it, nobody had ever thought that six carbon atoms could link to each other in any other way but in one straight line. By dreaming about six carbons in a hexagon or the cyclic nature of Benzene, as it is now popularly called, Kekule changed chemistry forever. Today when you read articles about how sleeping affects your hormones and therefore interferes with weight loss, spare a moment to thank him. Had it not been for his intuition about Benzene's true nature, you would have never figured out how lack of sleep leads to hormonal disturbances (your hormones have a lot of these cyclic structures) and how that affects your weight loss.

You may not believe that sleeping well awakens intuition, but you can continue reaping the benefits of better understood bio-chemistry. Did you just say, 'In your dreams'? Well, all I can say is, 'Sleep over it.' ☺

2. No booze before sleeping. Hello! I know you only sip the choicest wines and can go without drinking for years but only 'drink socially' to keep others company, or to keep people's mouths shut, or to not appear like a party pooper, or to just enjoy a romantic dinner or whatever.

(The funniest one I have heard is: 'Look I have to be a little tipsy to have sex with my husband. I can't stand him otherwise.') Yes, I know you are not exactly lying in a gutter every night because you are too drunk to go home. I know all that. I also know that you do vodka or the harder stuff only once in a while, and I know that you don't drink every day of the week. Yes, I know I am not talking to an alcoholic! But listen, I still think I should tell you about the alcohol and weight loss connection.

I have only been working for eleven years, and even in that span of time I have seen a dramatic rise in metabolic disorders in younger women, some younger than fifteen. The other thing that I have seen, is a dramatic rise in my clients' 'social drinking' and my gut tells me that there is a connection.

Alcohol is thought of as something that helps you fall asleep. Well, it's not entirely untrue. It does help you fall asleep, but prevents you from entering the REM or deep restorative stages of sleep. It's in these stages that our body carries out all the repair and restoration work of the body and mind. Okay, have you heard of the hypoxia or low oxygen levels and disrupted sleep? If you have ever been to Ladakh or know somebody who has been to Ladakh, then you have heard of altitude sickness or how they couldn't sleep for the first couple of nights? That's because the oxygen supply to the brain was not adequate so their sleep was interrupted and they kept waking up many times in the night. Alcohol does the exact same thing and is one of the reasons why you may not usually snore but will definitely snore on nights when you have had a drink or two. Snoring is a sign of poor or disturbed sleep. Now close your eyes and imagine somebody snoring next to you: is that somebody fat? We always associate snoring with fat people — why? Because disturbed sleep does lower your metabolism, making you stay fat.

Amongst many other things, alcohol reduces the levels of serotonin which helps you to feel calm and keeps your 'sugar cravings' under control. That glass of wine/vodka/rum/whatever it is, is again going to put you in the fight and flight mode and, equally bad, reduce your body's natural production of the growth hormone. It's going to create an environment in your body where you can't recover even though you slept like a log — come put your hands together and welcome the hangover. It's simply your hormones saying — I feel fatigued and dead tired.

Some more bad news? Well, if you have been working out regularly, then the alcohol destroys your endurance or stamina levels (you probably know that) and it reduces the levels of the hormone testosterone too. Say tata to toned muscles and strong bones and make friends with an expanding waist line. You really are a cool girl!

I sound like a bitch? Yeah, I feel like one too. Talking about alcohol makes me feel fatigued because that's the long-lasting feeling from booze, not the 'high', and tired women are always bitchy, right?

3. No dessert/pastry/sugar/tea/coffee — basically no stimulant — post sunset. Hmm… Now what can I tell you that you don't already know?

You know one of the things I absolutely hate is emails in my inbox from girly mags or Sunday newspapers asking me for examples of comfort food. Sample this:

Hi Rujuta,
Please send me very quickly answers to the following:
What are the comfort foods when feeling –

- *Bored*
- *Tired*
- *Lazy*
- *Cranky*
- *Fatigued*

Will appreciate your quick response. I need answers in detail by 3.30 p.m.

I had received this email at 1.30 p.m., and no, it was not from my boss or my mother-in-law; in fact it was nobody I had ever met/interacted with before. The only reason why this journo was throwing her weight around (according to me ninety per cent of journos are overweight) is because she worked for a 'most-read' paper. But even less popular papers/mags (and less-paid journos) will do this. **People who write about health have nothing to do with it. I think this also contributes to the rampant misinformation about food**, exercise and weight loss. What's more, they have little or no patience to understand anything about it.

Okay, I am done with whining and cribbing, so let's get to the point.

For starters, there is NO such thing as COMFORT FOOD. There definitely are depressed states of mind and fatigued bodies which look for a 'quick fix', but there's no way to quickly fix a tired mind and body and there are no quick answers to that email either. You know, when you see a woman dig into pastries or mithai or declare that she has a sweet tooth, then, well, then you can assume she is not getting enough action in bed! Oops, did I just say that? Yes, I did and I stand by it. The tongue is both a pleasure-giving and protecting organ. It tells you what's good for you and what's not, doesn't it? If you are eating something stale, it could be something beautifully presented in a five star hotel, the tongue won't be fooled by the eyes or the decor. It will declare, God! Is this dal last night's leftovers? And come on, I can guarantee that while you were digging into that sinful chocolate which overpowered your sense organs and the reasoning ability of your brain, your tongue declared — I shouldn't be eating this, or at least I should stop at two teaspoonfuls. See, the tongue protects, it tells you that overworking its pleasure centres is a crime. We have many pleasure centres, after all, right? Heard of genitals? Sorry, this book is for 'family reading' so let's put it this way: when the sexual organs are not nurtured it over-activates other pleasure centres. And eating too much sweet makes you dull, lethargic, unhealthy and fat and further reduces your chances of having sex.

The pleasure chakra

The swadhisthana chakra (remember it from the PCOD chapter? It's the chakra that not only controls or presides over your sexual desires, but also the desire to have more money or power) stays healthy and vibrant when one pursues money, power, sex meaningfully. So when I say 'not getting any action', I don't mean frequency, I mean purpose and meaning. Same goes with power and money — is it adding meaning to your life? If yes, you're in a good place.

What's more, the swadhisthana is involved with our creativity. The more labels we earn ('married', 'mother', 'working'), the less we pursue our hobbies — so no more Bharatnatyam, the sitar is fighting cobwebs, the badminton racket has been gifted to the bai, you no longer sing, not even in the bathroom, and you can't remember the last time you cooked for the sheer joy of it. So creativity is all stifled, drowning in worldly 'pleasures', leaving you no other option but to eat another chocolate post lunch! Tch tch. Grow up girls, let's make eating a pastry, mithai, chocolate a truly pleasurable activity where it doesn't send you on a guilt trip, not a minute after you eat, or hours later or the next morning.

The best way to ensure that eating mithai remains a sensory pleasure (and nothing else) is to not let it interfere with your sleep. Here's a simple formula you should byheart (ha ha) — Sleep well = no sugar cravings in the day. Eat sweets after dark = lack of good quality sleep = sugar cravings the next day = lack of good sleep. (The same applies for tea, coffee or any other stimulant; I've only used 'sweets' because we tend to succumb to that craving much more often.)

After sunset, the body uses a neurotransmitter called GABA to reduce adrenaline and increase serotonin and dopamine, basically reduces your feelings of agitation and alertness and increases feelings of calm and peace. Eating a sweet or drinking a cup of tea/coffee has the exact opposite effect, i.e. you are buzzing at night. This makes you fat yes, but also does not allow you to sleep well, which then reduces your recovery and destroys your immune function and also reduces the levels of GABA itself. The lower the levels of GABA, the more the feelings of anxiety or depression (one of the reasons why people suffer from nightmares the night after a late dinner and dessert), and when we are anxious or low or depressed what do we reach out for? Sorry, you don't win any medal for the answer. I'm hoping, though, that you now understand that it's best to eat your 'treat' by 4 p.m. or before it gets dark.

4. No compensation. Okay, I am not going to bore you with details but I just want to put one point across: SLEEP CANNOT BE COMPENSATED FOR. So if you tell yourself you 'compensate' for a week's lack of sleep by oversleeping on weekends, or you need a vacation to 'compensate' for all the late nights you've had, or that you need to go to mom's to sleep and 'compensate' for all the Diwali partying, you are seriously fooling yourself.

Sleep should be automatic, just like waking up should be automatic. (Automatic like breathing. You are breathing right now, right? I mean effortless = automatic.) When sleep and waking up is automatic or effortless, going to the loo, eating on time, eating right, looking fab, glowing skin, lustrous hair, pink nails, strong immune function, protection from lifestyle diseases, etc. is automatic or an absolute given. Following the first three sleep strategies will empower you to never ever needing to 'compensate' for sleep.

In fact, all the sleep strategies can be written as just one strategy: 'NO snooze' or ' NO alarm'. If you need an alarm to wake up, or worse need to put the alarm on the snooze mode, know that you are not respecting your body's need to sleep. Waking up fresh is not a dream, it's a reality and it's so worth working towards that reality.

Sleep and appetite

Leptin and ghrelin are hormones associated with your appetite. Leptin, secreted by fat cells, makes you feel full and asks you to stop eating further, while ghrelin, secreted by your GI tract, makes you feel hungry and urges you to eat. You need both to work well in order to stay fit, and these two need you to sleep well to function at their best. Not following the basics of the Sleep Strategies will lead to over-secretion of the hormone ghrelin in the night. You may think you're eating late or raiding the fridge just to kill time, but it's actually a result of excess ghrelin or the hunger hormone. Then you keep going to the loo, and again you think this is only because you are unable to sleep, but the reality is the leptin levels have gone down. Leptin works along with other calming hormones to ensure that you sleep undisturbed. But with low levels of calming hormones in the night, you experience what is often called as 'disturbed sleep' (sleeping but still not asleep), and it's this disturbance that stresses every part of your body and raises your body temperature so you go to the loo to pee in the hope of lowering the body temperature. What a waste of energies, na?

What's worse is, when you do this routinely, over months or years, the body gets resistant to leptin, which means you are producing adequate leptin but it can no longer do its work of giving you the satiety signal, asking you to stop eating or calming you down. So you get into a pattern of never feeling content or satisfied with whatever or no matter how much you eat. This leads to chronic overeating or eating something sweet post a meal. End result — more body fat than you can handle.

Chalo, have you understood how lack of sleep leads to an increase in episodes of overeating? Leptin resistance. To keep the appetite healthy (the ability to know when to eat, how much to eat and when to stop eating), you've got to ensure that ghrelin and leptin work, and to do that, all you've got do is sleep on time.

Bedroom etiquette

- Keep the bed a place exclusively to sleep, nothing else. Don't eat there. Keep the laptop, Blackberry, books away from it.
- Move your TV to another part of the house, and if that's not possible, switch it off while having dinner and one hour prior to bedtime.
- You need the body temperature to go down a bit to ensure a restful sleep, so keep the windows open and the bedroom well ventilated. If you need to use an AC, then set the temperature right so that you are not waking up to switch the AC off or fan on multiple times in the night.
- If you have trouble sleeping, avoid exercising after sunset because your body temperature goes up and metabolism picks up after exercise, which can keep you from falling asleep.
- Use curtains that allow sunlight to reach your bedroom so that your bio clock wakes you up naturally and activates your brain to pick up your metabolism and alertness levels too.
- Use natural and non-synthetic pillow covers, bed sheets, etc. Your skin should be able to breathe while sleeping. Synthetic covers or that satin lingerie/night dress can upset your body's temperature regulation and interfere with sleep. Also change the bed sheets every two days. (Our body drops dead cells during the night.)
- Burn a nice, relaxing aroma oil to soothe your senses. Open the windows of your bedroom often. Air and sun

bathe your bedding, don't just let it lie in the 'storage under the bed'.

- Bring back mosquito nets in place of chemical repellents.
- Above all, always go to bed at a fixed time. Okay, at least on most days of the week, sleep at a fixed hour.

IV

Relationship Strategies

If an Italian woman finds out her husband is having an affair, she will kill the other woman; a Spanish woman will kill her husband; and the Indian woman will kill herself!

–An old joke

See, an Indian woman will kill herself for just about anything, including losing weight. Uff! Teri adaa... Milk spilled? Bai extending leave without notice (yet again)? Father-in-law found too much masala in the food? Mother-in-law sulking because you left your cup on the table after drinking coffee? Mannu/Minni missed school bus by a whisker? Husband left dirty underwear for public display in the bathroom? Weight not budged in the last two weeks? God! I feel like killing myself! So the first thing we need to work on is our relationship with ourselves.

The need of the hour is for us to cultivate patience and forgiveness towards ourselves, to free ourselves from the unrealistic expectations we impose on ourselves, to learn to be our 'real' selves (not ideal). A REAL woman will put a hundred per cent effort towards all her responsibilities and KNOW that a hundred per cent effort is not equal to a hundred per cent result and an IDEAL woman doesn't exist. So stop chasing the unreal and get real. The real self is always happy, the unreal self is always searching for happiness and feeling lost. Also, getting fat and then unrealistically believing that losing weight will make you happy (or healthy) ... ha ha ha — what a cruel joke!

Obsessing with food and one's body, its shape, size and weight is a foolproof way of staying fat and unfit forever. Obsession with eating is now widely recognised as 'oral craving', a manifestation of some much deeper unresolved emotion. Ever noticed how eating too much at one time (often followed by long periods of starvation or 'detox') upsets your breathing? Invariably the breathing becomes faster, shorter, shallower, much like how it gets when you feel angry or upset. The breath is the link to the mind, when the breath is disturbed, so is the mind. When the breath is slow, soft, long, deep, the mind feels calm and at ease.

The Upanishads say that the diseases (getting fat is a disease dahlings, but NOT a crime) you create for yourself can be cured by yourself. And the Dalai Lama said, 'Problems cannot be resolved at the same levels of awareness that created them'. Samjha kya? You need to go from the level of being an ideal woman to a real woman if you must get healthier, happier (ya, ya to lose weight too).

So here are some strategies that will help you:

1. With power comes responsibility
2. Debugging sucks, testing rocks
3. Pain is our friend

1. With great power comes great responsibility — Spiderman said that. Now if the guy who goes around with a mask over his face can understand that, what's wrong with us? I mean, look at us women and the number of responsibilities we have. Do we have the power or access to resources which will help us fulfil our hajjar responsibilities — the access to education, healthcare, sanitation, family planning? If yes, then we must use this power to become more responsible towards ourselves. In a country like ours, you are a rare species if you said 'yes' to the above. Most of the Bharatiya naris will say 'no' or will have limited access depending on the whims of the current most powerful person in their lives (father/ husband/mother-in-law).

As a country, we have our problems, the cruellest being chronic hunger. Millions of Indians go hungry daily and a large number of them will die because of malnourishment. The biggest irony is that women like you and me, who have access (unlimited or limited) to resources will go hungry too, in the hope of losing weight. And if not totally hungry, we will invent so many fads and fears about food that we drive ourselves nuts: can't have peanuts; can't have rice at night; can't have puris; can't have ... can't have ... god! Food nourishes, lets you live, helps you carry out your responsibilities. And we've got that bonus, that we can study as long as we want, choose to reproduce when we want and have a bathroom which is not just clean, away from prying eyes but also practically designer. So now what? You have everything which ensures that you will NEVER be malnourished and yet you do everything that makes you malnourished. Yes, those vitamin B12, vitamin D3, iron, calcium deficiencies are screaming MALNOURISHMENT. Taking shots and popping pills doesn't work; being more responsible, getting more real and simple with food does.

How does this make its way to relationship strategies? How much and how well we eat is a sign of how much we value ourselves. All that power over reproduction, education, sanitation without self-worth is called... I don't know what it's called but, okay, undeserving, for the lack of a better word. Women are secondary citizens in our country but women like you and me have the power to at least at the personal level end the discrimination. Eat, and eat bindaas and at the time you need food, not after children are sent to school, dabba is made for husband, father-in-law finishes eating, etc. Get it?

2. Debugging sucks, testing rocks (seen in the Google India, Hyderabad office loo). In the IT industry, if there's a problem with the program you've written, then you need to rewrite or recreate that program — a huge hassle and a time-consuming task. The process is called debugging. A much more effective thing to do is 'testing': check for everything that can go wrong and make a provision to ensure that it doesn't. Testing may appear time-consuming, but in fact it saves not just time, but also a lot of hassle. What's more, it makes you look smart. You've already checked and rechecked for all failures and plugged all the loopholes — what a smart girl you make!

Now use this great strategy and apply it to all your relationships, including that with food. So you decided to eat right, what can go wrong? You may not find dahi at 4 p.m.; you may run out of poha or oil to make breakfast; you forgot to take that calcium tablet at night; your colleagues may eat all your peanuts; you will only be offered biscuits or at best a sandwich at that working lunch meeting. So then what? If you start debugging or fixing the problem after it has already occurred, it sucks. Since you are one hell of a rockstar, or at least want to look like one, you must anticipate everything that can go wrong before it does and have back-up options; it's called testing and it's rocking.

Initially you may need to do testing on a daily basis, later weekly and over a period of time it will become an integral part of you. You won't even notice that you are testing, just like you don't even notice that you ate lunch late again today. Some tips for testing:

- Before going to sleep, decide what you will be eating for breakfast and check if the kitchen has everything you need to make it. Make a checklist: gas – check, poha – check, oil – check, herbs, spices, masala dabba – check, coconut – check, etc.
- Fix the days when you will go to your local bhaji market and buy veggies for not more than three days. Don't use the fridge as a store room and use a cloth bag to ferry your stuff. Walk to the market: that way you can burn calories and save parking time and petrol costs.
- If all you get is biscuits for meetings, bark (dogs eat biscuits) at the HR/management. Employee welfare means access to nutritious food, not coffee machines, biscuits and chips in the pantry and a smoking booth.
- Ensure that your handbag has two food options in it at all times.
- Keep your vitamins and minerals in a place where you can see them, that way you won't forget to take them. Investing in a fancy pill box works well too: that way you can have it in your handbag at all times.
- Decide at the breakfast table what your 4-6 p.m. meal is going to be and arrange it before stepping out of the house. Ya baby, you are not alone; we all eat wrong

during that golden two-hour period. Actually we should be eating dinner around that time.

3. Pain is our friend. It tells us that something is wrong and needs to be corrected. When the children's homework, husband's TV viewing, mother-in-law, friend's bickering, standing for a long time becomes a pain, it's actually shouting CHANGE. In our current relationship with ourselves, we have learnt to put up with or brave the pain. Eating too late in the night, drinking more than two cups of tea/coffee in the day, grabbing breakfast, skipping lunch, and dabaoing dinner is painful (whether you do it once or all the time) — but do we change? No, we are such lazy girls that we'd rather blame our relationships with other people than change our own eating habits. 'What to do, my husband comes back home so late.' You must have heard that before, right? Why do you eat so late? My husband comes back so late! God! But you are at home, didn't you see yourself? Are you invisible? Become visible in your own eyes, allow your most basic need to eat to become visible, so visible that it's difficult to not see that you are hungry while carrying out your 'responsibilities' or while trying to get 'thin'.

4. Okay, stomach this: **the most intimate relationship you will ever have is with food**. No? Why? What's the first thing you did when you were born? Breathe? And then? Had milk? Well, do you know that your lungs are actually an off-shoot of your gastrointestinal tract? So even before making provision for you to breathe, Mother Nature made provision for you to eat. Your intestines are supposed to be your first point of contact with the world, in a way your intestines surround you and allow you to interact with both the outside and inside worlds.

Way too often we use food as a means of filling a void that we may be experiencing, to seek love, approval or intimacy, but all this leads to is filling the body with excess fat which reduces its mobility, stability and utility. Ironically, it actually reduces our ability to give and receive love, approval and intimacy. Food, often referred to as dravya in our ancient texts, is meant to heal, strengthen and nourish the body. And the body is meant for a higher purpose, that of achieving the maximum human potential, that of enlightenment.

We have our bodies, just like we have bed sheets, a pair of jeans, etc., but at no point do we *become* the bed sheet or jeans, right? We accept that they are useful for the purpose that we have them for, and understand that we can use them as long as we take care of them and no matter how well we take care of them, one day you will give up the bed sheet.

The food you eat is your way of internalising (and becoming a part of) the universe. So what do you want to internalise? The fresh warmth of 'home-cooked, grown-with-love fruits, veggies, grains, dals, legumes, milk (hey! I am thinking that you are going to buy into my "farm mother" concept), eaten in peace, digested with calm, absorbed with care, assimilated with responsibility and excreted with sensibility' food? Or the 'well-packaged (low-fat, fibre-enriched, fortified with calcium or some such "eye ball grabber" on the cover), made for the convenience-seeking, gullible buyer, eaten — sorry grabbed — on-the-go, digested with distraction, absorbed minimally, assimilated with stress and excreted with strain' food?

As with all things in life, the choice is totally yours.

5

Things You Should Know

1. How to deal with hair loss, breakouts and more
2. Traditional vs packaged cereal breakfasts
3. Planning your weekly exercise calendar

1. How to deal with hair loss, breakouts and more
Micronutrient deficiencies can bring about a whole lot of physiological changes in our body, leading to a compromise in our hormonal health. These changes often show on our skin and hair, but small corrections in our diet can change that. Listed below are some examples.

Note: Hidden hunger is what micro-nutrient deficiency is called in populations that have enough to eat but still suffer from inadequate levels of certain nutrients — Iron, vitamin D, B12, etc.

Condition	Doing this?	Facts	Action
Hair loss, split ends and dandruff	Consuming low or zero-fat products — from milk to cheese to yogurt to cutting out dairy altogether. Adding fibre to rotis, or eating cereals marketed as fibre-rich, even picking biscuits that have fibre. Avoiding wholesome meals, especially at night. Eg: Instead of dal-rice-sabzi eating only dal and sabzi.	Deficiency in protein, essential fat and zinc (caused by low-calorie, low-carb diets, medication) prevents natural hair growth and makes the hair look dull, frizzy, dry.	Good hair comes from eating homemade white butter, tadka on dals, ghee on rotis, regular oiling of hair, coconut in chutneys and rice on your plates. So check for what's missing and bring it back.

Condition	Doing this?	Facts	Action
Breakouts	Avoiding dinners and bingeing late at night. Nibbling on a chocolate or even feeling like eating one post lunch or dinner. Picking low cal or 'healthy' versions of pastries and desserts. Alcohol, even if it's only socially, or just a glass of wine.	Not eating anything for a long time and snacking on sweet stuff (even if it's free of sugar/fat, etc.) impairs nutrient absorption from the food we eat. Alcohol, even in small amounts, makes it really difficult for the gut to hold on to the friendly bacteria, which further drives you to eat processed, very sweet or salty stuff.	The skin looks good when it receives all the nourishment from food. For that you need to eat local and what is in season. Avoid anything that comes out of a box. To rebuild the gut-friendly bacteria and heal breakouts, try these three power foods: banana every morning, dahi-rice at least twice a week, and yes, water, plenty of it, through the day.
Pigmentation and patchy skin	Juices and other detox stuff every now and then. Switched to some heart-healthy oil and given up on traditional oils like groundnut, mustard, coconut. Staying away from ghee. Skipping breakfast often or having a long gap between rising and the first meal.	Pigmentation on the skin is often a result of micronutrient deficiency, mostly those of minerals like iron, calcium and zinc. And also those of fat-soluble vitamins like D and E.	Make nuts, specially cashews, an essential part of your diet. They are a great source of minerals, fibre and essential fat, all of which work wonders for the skin. Eat ragi or nachni roti twice every week to meet your nutrient needs and don't forget the laddoos in winter. The ones that come with goond, aliv, etc.
Water retention	Staying in an AC environment for a long time. Not drinking enough water. Eating breads or packaged cereals. Straining on the toilet and having laxatives often.	Excess salt, poor quality protein, dehydration and loss of vitamin B often shows up as bloating or water retention. The fact that it often comes with constipation only makes it worse.	Drink water and make a conscious effort to eat your dals and legumes. Sprout them, cook them well and eat them with your rice or roti — that's when you get all the goodness you need to keep the bloating down. Switch to unrefined salts (those that retain potassium and other minerals too) for at least one meal a day. And get some fresh air.

Condition	Doing this?	Facts	Action
Bags and dark circles under the eyes	Tons of screen time and very little me time. Big dinners and skipped lunches. Almost no fresh fruit consumption through the week.	Overall a sign of poor lifestyle: one that's low on nourishment, exercise and sleep.	Ensure that you are not on a gadget at least one hour prior to bed time. Eat a wholesome meal by 6 p.m. and plan it a week in advance. Poha, ghee-jaggery-roti, seasonal fruit are all good options. And don't forget to make exercise an integral part of your life.

2. Starting the day right: a comparison of traditional and on-the-go breakfast options

A good beginning is ninety per cent of the weight-loss battle won! So begin your day with a hot, homemade, traditional nashta. You'll see, from the chart below, how a traditional Indian breakfast beats your 'low-calorie' cereal/milk any day.

Most of the homemade breakfast options given below can be cooked in fifteen minutes (provided the raw material needed for it is procured and kept ready). Although this requires some time off from your 'busy' schedule, it's an investment that is surely worth it because it is absolutely essential for a fit and toned body — something that adds value to your life and well-being.

These are approximate values for a healthy and happy serving: not too much to make you feel stuffed, not too little that you're left unsatisfied. ☺

Food item	Calories (kcals)	Protein (g)	CHO (g)	Fat (g)	Iron (mg)	Calcium (mg)	Fibre (g)
Aloo paratha	400	7.6	65	10.1	3.42	38.8	9.2

Nutrient composition: Homemade aloo paratha with ghee is a wholesome meal with a high satiety value and rich in essential fat (ghee). Aloo is a good source of B6 (pyridoxine), vitamin C, potassium, manganese, essential amino acid tryptophan and phytonutrients — carotenoids, flavonoids. It is also a good source of natural dietary fibre in the adequate amount required (which will not interfere with the absorption of vitamins and minerals).

Spices like ajwain help improve digestion as well as have anti-flatulence properties.

Cosmetic use: Will prevent you from feeling bloated.

Food Item	Calories (kcals)	Protein (g)	CHO (g)	Fat (g)	Iron (mg)	Calcium (mg)	Fibre (g)
Idli/ Dosa + sambhar + chutney	334	12	54	7	2.09	98.5	10.58

Nutrient composition: Idli/Dosa + sambhar + chutney is a complete meal with an appropriate balance of carbs, protein, fat, vitamins and minerals. Idli/dosa is a rich source of B12, along with essential fats. Being a cereal–pulse combination, it has all the essential amino acids. Spices like turmeric and mustard add to the nutrient value of this meal. Mustard is rich in selenium and therefore has a strong antioxidant quality. Turmeric, which is a natural colouring and flavouring agent, is also an antiseptic, and has anti-inflammatory and healing properties.

Cosmetic use: Helps dark circles and puffy eyes.

Food Item	Calories (kcals)	Protein (g)	CHO (g)	Fat (g)	Iron (mg)	Calcium (mg)	Fibre (g)
Poha	290	6.45	42.6	9.46	7.1	54.9	6.28

Nutrient composition: Poha is the most common breakfast option, and is an ideal meal in itself. Rice flakes are a good source of iron, and if you squeeze a lemon into it, you will improve on your iron absorption as well. Traditionally peanuts are added to it, which contain MUFA, essential amino acids — tryptophan, B vitamins — niacin, biotin, folate. It is also rich in oleic acid (the essential fat found in olive oil as well), along with high concentrations of antioxidants, especially polyphenols. Spices such as curry leaves and mustard are natural flavouring agents, which improve the digestive function by increasing salivary secretion and secretion of digestive juices, improving the function of the small intestine and hence enhancing nutrient absorption.

Cosmetic use: Will get you closer to a flat tummy.

Food Item	Calories (kcals)	Protein (g)	CHO (g)	Fat (g)	Iron (mg)	Calcium (mg)	Fibre (g)
Suji halwa	**360**	**1.56**	**30**	**20.12**	**0.26**	**4.2**	**1.87**

Nutrient composition: Suji halwa is the most loved as well as the most avoided breakfast option ☺. This is the best way to start your day, if you are a sweet lover. The richness of homemade ghee, blended well with semolina and sugar, will give you a nutrient-dense meal — all your essential fats, MUFA and B-complex vitamins. Essential fats will help lubricate your joints, lower your sweet cravings, improve your fat metabolism, reduce your stubborn fat stores, give you a feeling of satiety and will calm your nerves and senses. B-complex vitamins will help improve your carbohydrate metabolism, improve the utilisation of carbs, proteins and fat from your meal. (Even though suji halwa is not high in fibre, the ghee present in it acts as a natural laxative and promotes peristalsis as well.)

Cosmetic use: Leads to soft, smooth and supple skin.

Food Item	Calories (kcals)	Protein (g)	CHO (g)	Fat (g)	Iron (mg)	Calcium (mg)	Fibre (g)
Poori bhaji	425	4.6	43.6	25.1	1.95	24.4	5.45

Nutrient composition: Poori bhaji is a traditional breakfast in the east (where it's called luchi aloo), but is considered unhealthy because of its 'high fat' content. Poori bhaji is a wholesome meal which has a good satiety value. It is a good source of vitamins (B-complex and vitamin C), minerals and phytonutrients. Spices and herbs like cumin seeds, ginger and coriander help improve the palatability, have therapeutic properties and also help improve our metabolism (by aiding digestion). Cumin seeds (jeera) are a good source of iron and manganese. Jeera helps keep our immune system healthy, boosts proper digestion and nutrient assimilation. Ginger is regarded as an excellent carminative (a substance which promotes the elimination of intestinal gas) and intestinal spasmolytic (a substance which relaxes and soothes the intestinal tract), and has an anti-inflammatory and anti-carcinogenic action. Coriander has essential oils which have anti-rheumatic and anti-arthritic properties, is an effective diuretic (helps regulate blood pressure) and plays a role in stimulating the digestive juices and peristalsis.

Cosmetic use: Will prevent dandruff and dry skin.

Food Item	Calories (kcals)	Protein (g)	CHO (g)	Fat (g)	Iron (mg)	Calcium (mg)	Fibre (g)
Processed commercial cereals with skimmed milk	220	7.9	29.5	8	1.5	180	3.3

Nutrient composition: Processed/commercial cereals with skimmed milk, which is now supposed to be the 'ideal on-the-go' convenience breakfast option is not as healthy compared to your traditional breakfast options.

You don't really feel satisfied with the serving size mentioned on the box (30 g), and it leaves you feeling hungrier and makes your sweet cravings shoot up through the day. So even though it is considered a 'low-calorie breakfast', you actually end up eating a SMALL chotu piece of chocolate post-lunch or a pastry post-dinner. This is because when you start your day off with a meal that doesn't give you the kind of satiety and nutrients that you require (after a night of fasting because you are sleeping), you will definitely end up eating much more through the day (your body needs to make up for the calorie deficit). And to top it, all commercial/packaged cereals are loaded with preservatives, artificial colouring and flavouring agents, which not only hamper your nutrient absorption but also compromises the functioning of your digestive tract and strips you of your existing nutrient stores.

Cosmetic use: Minimum investment of time.

3. Planning your weekly exercise calendar

Here is a suggested plan:

	Weeks 1 – 8	Week 8 onwards	Note
Day 1	Strength training – Basic workout as per the Beginner's workout given below	Strength training – Upper body as per the Intermediate workout given below	Focus on: - Specific warm-up - Big muscles - Compound movements
Day 2	Yoga asana	Yoga asana	Learn from a good teacher from one of the traditional schools of yoga like Iyengar, Mysore, Sivananda, Bihar, etc.
Day 3	Hobby	Hobby	Pick up a hobby which you have been wanting to pursue but haven't so far. Keeps your creative side alive.
Day 4	Cardio – 20 minutes	Strength training – Lower body as per the Intermediate workout given below	For more details on progressive overload in cardio and strength training, read *Don't Lose Out, Work Out!*
Day 5	Rest	Cardio – 20 to 30 minutes	Choose from running, cycling, swimming, elliptical. Progressive overload each week.
Day 6	Yoga asana	Yoga asana	If it's not possible to join a class or learn from a teacher, you can refer to *Illustrated Light on Yoga* by BKS Iyengar and follow it at home.
Day 7	Rest	Rest	Often neglected but a very crucial aspect of exercise.

Beginner's plan

Exercise	Target muscle group	Sets	Reps
Leg extension	Quads	1	12-15
Leg press	Quads, Glutes, Hamstrings	2	12-15
Leg curl	Hamstring	1	12-15
Adductor/Abductor	Inner thigh/Outer thigh	1	12-15
Lat pull down	Lats (back)	1-2	12-15
Seated row	Lats, Traps (back)	1-2	12-15
Hyper extension	Lower back	1	12-15
Dumbbell/Bar press	Chest and shoulders	2	12-15
Pec dec/fly	Chest	1-2	12-15
Side laterals	Shoulder	1	12-15
Dumbbell curl	Bicep	1	12-15
Tricep push down	Triceps	1	12-15

Intermediate plan

Exercise	Target muscle group	Sets	Reps
Lower body			
Leg extension	Quads	1	12-15
Leg press	Quads, Glutes, Hamstring	2	12-15
Leg curl	Hamstring	1	12-15
Adductor/Abductor	Inner thigh/Outer thigh	1	12-15
Upper body			
Lat pull down	Lats (back)	1-2	12-15
Seated row	Lats, Traps (back)	1-2	12-15
Hyper extension	Lower back	1	12-15
Dumbbell/Bar press	Chest and shoulders	2	12-15
Pec dec/fly	Chest	1-2	12-15
Side laterals	Shoulder	1	12-15
Dumbbell curl	Bicep	1	12-15
Tricep push down	Triceps	1	12-15

6

FAQs: Ten Questions from Readers

Name	Topic
Richa Bhake Ghatole	Hypothyroid and lethargy
Rachna Prasad	PCOD and hostel food
Anshu Sharma	Supplements for PCOD-thyroid
Neha Karda	PCOD and weight-training
Divya Ram	PCOD and refined sugar
Sreevidya Subramanian	Hypothyroid and hair loss
Neeti Gupta Kanungo	Hypothyroid and medication
Durva Shastri	Yoga for PCOD
Pratik Agarwal for his sister	PCOD and weight gain
Anushri Jana	PCOD and facial hair

Q: *As a hypothyroid patient, I am often overcome by lethargy. How can I break through this to get moving and exercise? Please don't say, 'Just get off your lazy ass'; it is not that simple. I hope there are small exercises that can just get me going.*

Also, is hypothyroid genetic? My mom and her two sisters have it as well.

–Richa Bhake Ghatole, Vadodra

A: There are small steps that one can take towards feeling energetic and enthusiastic about exercise. But before that, not feeling up to exercise is not so much about hypothyroid as it is about the lack of adequate amounts of vitamin D. A vitamin D deficiency and hypothyroid is a bit like the chicken and egg situation: it's tough to tell which came first but they both exist together. You are more likely to have gotten your hypothyroid from a vitamin D deficiency than from your mom or aunts.

Gyan apart, what can you do about it? Four things:

1. Include essential fats like homemade ghee and coconut in your diet. The essential fatty acids you get from these are important for vitamin D assimilation in the body; it's a fat-soluble vitamin, remember? Adequate vitamin D levels help the thyroid glands function at their optimum level.
2. Eat a handful of cashews every day. Rich in micro-minerals and iron, cashews help the body feel better in terms of energy levels. Iron is an integral part of haemoglobin and plays a critical role in the oxygenation of tissues and prevents lethargy from setting in.
3. Go gadget-free at least one hour prior to bedtime because, finally, sleep is the biggest hormone regulator. And without good sleep you can almost never wake up fresh enough to work out.
4. Lastly, know that it takes only about 150 minutes a week of exercise to keep the metabolic diseases, including thyroid, at bay. So begin with a target of one hour a week. Put that in your calendar; days, time and type of workout for every week. Follow it through and know that every extra minute is a bonus. From there you can build it up slowly to 150 minutes a week. Details in *Don't Lose Out, Work Out!*

Q: *My daughter has PCOD and lives in a hostel, so managing her diet is tough. What advice would you give to manage this condition better?*

–Rachna Prasad

A: Well, Rachna, what I have seen is that it's girls who have stayed away from home at an early stage who are at a much bigger risk of developing hormonal imbalances than those who have lived at homes with a kitchen and with their mothers to nurture them. I especially find that hostels and a competitive environment are a lethal combination for hormones. Anyway, we can't stop living in hostels, but we can surely stop ourselves from ruining our health. I would suggest the following:

1. Always ensure that your girl has a stock of dry fruits and that she starts her day with a handful of those before reaching out for some caffeine drink (tea/coffee/energy drink).
2. Advocate limiting tea/coffee intake to max three cups a day, and to never have it a) In place of a meal, b) First thing in the morning and c) Last thing in the night.
3. Cut down on aerated drinks, including their diet or zero cal versions; energy drinks like Red/Blue/Yellow Bull etc.; and protein drinks like Bournvita/Complan/Horlicks/Protinex, etc. Too much sugar and too industrialised, best avoided.
4. Give her a box of ladoos — besan/rava/aliv/goond, take your pick for every season — and tell her it's a great mid-meal, post-lunch or post-breakfast snack. Meets her mineral and energy requirements, and she won't be reaching out for those chocolates late at night.

5. Stop all instant, packaged foods/snacks and install an electric induction plate in her room on which she can cook dal-chawal. Urge her to cook at least once a week as a long-term weight management strategy.
6. Send homemade ghee and tell her to add a teaspoon on as many meals as possible, and if that is not possible, to have at least one teaspoon every single day by itself. The short-chain fatty acids keep the intestinal mucus healthy and ensures good digestion. And yes, it's a beautiful weight-loss aid too.
7. Don't ask if she is studying; instead ask if she is playing. Ideally it should be at least ninety minutes a day, and if that's not happening, then a minimum of an hour a day. So let academics and project reports wait; play and exercise should come first. Grades don't bring health or hormonal balance, but active play does.
8. Lastly, do tell her that more than one late night a week is going to come in the way of her waist and her jeans. And if she must stay up, then good meal options are makhana/nuts/homemade chivda/bread + butter/milk with sugar or honey (with no additives)/peanuts.

That's a long list, and I hope it helps.

Q: *Hey Rujuta, what are the must-have supplements if someone is suffering from these lifestyle disorders?*

–Anshu Sharma, Melbourne

A: Anshu, a supplement does just that, supplements. What is critical here is an overall positive and committed attitude towards one's health. So this is going to be a repetition of what I have been saying but here goes:

1. Eating fresh: Food that is local, seasonal and regional is the key here. Buy fresh food, ensure that it is in season and cook food using recipes that you inherited from your mother. That's a better way to eat healthy food, better than following any good-looking chef on social media or googling the latest trend, be it kale or quinoa.
2. Exercise: Work out 150 minutes per week, without fail, and plan for this a week in advance. That way you won't prioritise other stuff and people before your gym/ workout time.
3. Sleep: Regulate bedtime and wake-up time, as sleep quality influences our ability to digest food and even to eliminate toxins.

There is no such thing as a must-have supplement; the above three are the only must-haves. And the following three help when the above three are in place:

1. Vitamin B-complex with an extra strength of vitamin B12. Aids carbohydrate metabolism and prevents dullness.
2. Calcium — important to keep the bone density and prevent cramps and aches during periods.
3. Essential fatty acids — not really important to take it in a pill or powder form, but that teaspoon of homemade ghee at every meal works wonders for insulin sensitivity and your skin; it even prevents acne. God bless ghee!

Q: *PCOD is a condition where there are more male hormones in the body. You've said weight-training won't pump women up like it does men because their hormones are different. Does weight-training for women with PCOD pump them* *up because they have more testosterone? My dietician said a big no to weight training for women with PCOD because their bodies become like men, owing to the presence of this hormone. Please resolve this confusion for me.*

–Neha Karda, Hyderabad

A: Classically, PCOD is about insulin resistance and from there starts the entire imbalance, whether it's in our estrogen to testosterone ratios or high prolactin levels, or high homocysteine levels. Weight-training, my dear, regulates the testosterone levels in the body but, and that's a big but, you have got to do it the right way. That's like saying that flying to Delhi from Hyderabad will take you to Delhi but you have to be on the right flight, you can't be on a flight to Kolkata and then say, 'I flew but I am still not in Delhi'. Getting the drift?

Sports scientists have now proved beyond reasonable doubt that it is the muscle quality that determines how well we regulate blood sugar and therefore can prevent hormonal disorders and associated weight gain. Muscle quality is defined as maximum force production per unit of muscle mass. Basically science is saying that being strong is going to make us more like women than like men. So you must not just weight-train, you must consistently work at lifting heavy, and then simply trust good old physiology to keep the hormones, weight and blood sugar in check. Read *Don't Lose Out, Work Out!* for weight-training routines and more information.

Most dieticians and doctors are unaware and misinformed about using strength-training as a lifestyle intervention, and instead focus heavily on calorie control and drugs. Which is not just incorrect but very boring and over a period of time just reduces your confidence to a number on the weighing scale and makes you rely heavily on drugs. Please be informed that one of the side-effects of weight-training is increased sex drive ;).

Q: *Is there a direct link to refined sugar and PCOD or is it just another bit of misinformation floating around?*

–Divya Ram

A: Sugar, Divya, is one of the panch amrits of India, along with milk, ghee, curd and honey, or banana if you are a south Indian. Apna table sugar or cane sugar (like Starbucks calls it), sugar that comes from sugarcane, is good, very good, life-saving medicine really. One of the reasons why it's a panch amrit is because it prevents ageing, more specifically prevents those fine lines that start showing on the side of our eyes and around our eyes. Glycolic acid — an alpha hydroxy acid or AHA like the cosmetic products call it — present in sugarcane prevents this skin damage, works at rebuilding collagen tissue and keeps us looking fresh and beautiful.

Sugar in all forms is good: chew sugarcane, drink its freshly-crushed juice, have it as jaggery or as plain crystalline sugar. Typically, we use sugar in summer as it is cooling in nature, and jaggery in winter as it's heating in nature. So feel free to add sugar to your tea/coffee, sherbets and even home-made sweets — the laddoos, the halwas, etc.

Also, know that even the USFDA updated its guidelines recently to warn against the use of sweeteners as a weight-loss or hormone-regulating aid, because of all of the side-effects associated with it.

So no, it's not sugar, it's how you use it. Prevent its consumption through that piece of chocolate, the cookie you nibbled mindlessly, the cereal you bought for weight-loss, and the packaged juice you drink as a healthy snack. Sugar is like that crush you have on your colleague: if you marry him and take him home, it's going to be a disaster, but flirting in small amounts daily will spice up your life ☺.

Note: Even world health regulatory bodies, like the American Heart Association, says six to nine teaspoons of sugar daily is okay.

Q: *Hi Rujuta, I have hypothyroid, but in the last two months, I have started losing a lot of hair. It's very disturbing and depressing. I don't know what to do and how to stop it.*

–Sreevidya Subramanian, Germany

A: Oh yes, that can be quite a disturbing sight — a bunch of hair after you wash it or the one that's on the pillow every morning. However, once you regulate the delivery of amino acids (proteins) and iodine to your body, than not just hair, even your thyroid gland will feel much better. Here are a few things you can do to prevent hair fall:

1. Eat rice. I know you must have been told not to eat rice, but hand-pounded or single-polished rice (looks more white than brown in colour) retains the right amount of vitamin B, minerals and fibre in it. These along with the branched chain amino acids found in rice promotes good hair growth.

2. Paneer (or fresh cheese since you live in Germany), milk or nuts — one of them must be a part of your daily diet. It not just provides a good profile of amino acids but is also a good source of essential fatty acids which is essential for the absorption of vitamin D, which regulates the thyroid hormone and in turn promotes hair health.
3. Make coconut part of your diet, either as chutney or while cooking. When it's tough to find a coconut, get an avocado. The fats found in coconut promote hair growth and fat loss. Kate Hudson recently said that her glow is because of coconut — basically even Hollywood is now taking your grandmom's advice seriously.
4. Use unrefined or Himalayan salt while cooking — it is rich in micro-minerals and provides iodine to the body.
5. Apply coconut oil to your hair and often. At least once a week heat coconut oil and add methi seeds to it. Let it cool and then massage it into your scalp. Let it stay for at least half an hour before washing it off.

Q: *Hi Rujuta. I have hypothyroidism and am on medication — 100 mcg of Thyronorm. My thyroid test readings always fall in the normal range, yet I still feel most of the symptoms I did before I started medication, particularly bloating and weight gain. No doctor has given me a good reason for this. Please advise.*

–Neeti Gupta Kanungo, Delhi

A: That's the thing Neeti, most of us get put on medication a tad bit aggressively. By that I mean that we are put on medication the minute one blood test shows that TSH is higher than 5 and in some cases just higher than 3, even when t4 and t3 readings are in range, and also the lipid profile or the glycaemic control is measured as HbA1c.

We start the medication in full faith but fail to correct the lifestyle factors that caused the TSH to go up in the first place. What is required really is extensive counselling for a complete lifestyle overhaul and that starts with one step at a time. This is what I recommend you start doing to beat the bloating and lose the weight:

1. Start your day with a banana, the local one. The micro-minerals help keep the bloating down and have the right nutrients to act as a pre-biotic. Basically works at helping you retain the gut-friendly bacteria and in the assimilation of vitamin B12. So you never run out of energy or feel big on the stomach.
2. Try nachni kheer or ragi satva for breakfast at least two to three times a week, or roll it into a ladoo and have it as a mid-meal. The homemade ghee and ragi combination is a great way to improve vitamin D assimilation, directly related to thyroid health, and also increases bone mineral density which in turn will help keep the body volume/size down.
3. Nap every afternoon for about fifteen to twenty minutes post lunch. Great for recovery and helps improve fat-burning. The key is to nap, not sleep or lay around for hours together. Works like magic at killing the sugar craving too.
4. Weight-train — I cannot say this often enough. But this is one overlooked and undervalued lifestyle intervention which works better than the pill. Do it

consistently and long enough, it will help you get rid of the meds too.

Q: *I've consulted a hell of a lot of gynaecologists to cure my PCOD but in vain. They subscribe heavy medicines that have got side-effects. But I have started performing yoga and try to follow your principles. My question to you is — is yoga enough to cure my PCOD? Will it ever get cured? Thanks in advance.*

–Durva Shastri, Ahmedabad

A: Just this morning, as I hung upside down on ropes in my Iyengar yoga class, my teacher said, see you do this and you will never need a sonography, blood report or medicines. Padma Vibhushan BKS Iyengar, a legend celebrated world over, with multiple scientific papers in medical journals inspired by his work on the therapeutic effect of asanas on all conditions, especially lifestyle disorders, is almost unknown, or his method is not even explored in the effort to keep healthy. Asanas should actually be our go-to option every time we feel that our cycles are off the mark. More specifically, classical schools of yoga like the Iyengar school, Sivananda school, Bihar School of Yoga, Mysore school, etc. (details on how to choose your yoga school in *Don't Lose Out, Work Out!*), with teachers who are guided by a strong sense of ethics and deep-rooted practice.

Eating right and doing consistent, well-rounded asana practice can help you not just provide the right nourishment, oxygenation and circulation to your reproductive system but will help you feel lighter and more energetic too. By that I mean a regular, effortless period without acne, back pain or irritability. Good enough?

In short, yoga is not India's biggest export to the world for nothing. It has the ability to alleviate everything that leads to a less-than-perfect or un-harmonious existence for humankind.

Q: *I have an old history of PCOS and did my USG last year. It seems normal. My cycles are also normal, but the days shift every month and I have also gained weight since last year. Please advise.*

–Pratik Agrawal, for his sister

A: There are a few things here that you should consider:

1. Weight gain is not always because of hormones — in fact, most often it is not. It is due to our lifestyle factors: diet, exercise, sleep and even relationships. Consider what has changed on all these fronts before thinking that this is due to hormones.
2. The period moving by a few days or even a week is totally cool, nothing abnormal about that. However, if it's painful, crampy and makes you moody, then that is what you need to address, not the date. The chapter on PCOD in this book covers it in detail.
3. Yogic belief is that healthy and therefore fertile women get their periods during the increasing phase of the moon. Sickness, ageing and stress can make periods come during the waning moon, a sign of low fertility too.

4. Sometimes it's just something as simple as vitamin B12 that changes the period cycle. So make sure that you are eating plenty of fresh food, having a glass of chaas at least once a day, and including homemade pickle in your diet.

Q: *I have controlled my PCOD by following your book since last year. A big thanks to you. I have improved a lot in terms of insulin insensitivity and lost around ten kilos. I feel so much better now. But I have terrible PMS and hirsutism is a problem. Please guide.*

–Anushri Jana, Pune

A: Well done, Anushri! It's really good to know that you followed the strategies and helped your insulin get more sensitive and lost weight. The effort to make those consistent changes is entirely yours and to your credit, so don't thank me, instead accept my gratitude for sharing your journey with all of us.

For PMS and hirsutism, here are a few things you can do:

PMS:

- Double up your calcium a week before your period so that you don't get the aches or cramps.
- Start your day with a banana to keep the bloating and sugar cravings at bay.
- Eat a handful of kaju as a mid-meal snack to keep the mood swings and emotions under control.

Hirsutism/Facial hair:

Hirsutism or facial hair is also genetic and if there's one factor which can help us reduce it, it is an improved body composition. For that you basically need to keep up with all the things that you are already doing that have improved your insulin sensitivity. Insulin sensitivity helps us keep our other hormones in check. Androgen or male hormones in levels higher than normal are associated with the hair growth. Do the following for further improving insulin sensitivity:

- Strength train at least twice a week to improve muscle quality, which in turn improves insulin sensitivity.
- Practice yoga asanas twice a week, sincerely and fearlessly — specially the inversions and back bends. These often get ignored by women but are critical for keeping our male and female hormones in the right proportion.
- Make home-made white butter a part of your regular diet to help with good assimilation of fat-soluble vitamins — especially A, E and D — involved in keeping the skin supple and glowing.
- Try the home remedy of besan, malai and turmeric as a facial application, which is known to both reduce and lighten hair growth.
- Last but not the least, know that it takes time for changes to come through in their full glory. Acknowledge every step in the right direction as progress and keep at it with patience and diligence.

All the best!